ULTIMATE
YOU

ULTIMATE YOU

A 4-PHASE TOTAL BODY MAKEOVER FOR WOMEN WHO WANT MAXIMUM RESULTS

JOE DOWDELL, CSCS,
and Brooke Kalanick, ND, MS

RODALE

Rodale books may be purchased for business or promotional use or for special sales. For information, please write to: Special Markets Department, Rodale Inc., 733 Third Avenue, New York, NY 10017

Photographs by Thomas MacDonald
Book design by Christina Gaugler

Library of Congress Cataloging-in-Publication Data

Dowdell, Joe.
    Ultimate you : a 4-phase total body makeover for women who want maximum results / Joe Dowdell and Brooke Kalanick.
        p.   cm.
    ISBN-13 978–1–60529–627–2   hardcover
    ISBN-10 1–60529–627–9   hardcover
    1. Physical fitness for women.   2. Women—Nutrition.   I. Kalanick, Brooke.   II. Title.
GV482.D69 2010
613.7'045—dc22   2010005117

Distributed to the trade by Macmillan

2   4   6   8   10   9   7   5   3   1   hardcover

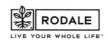

For all the women taking the time,
energy, and dedication to exercise,
eat well, and care for themselves—
here's to achieving your Ultimate You.

Contents

CHAPTER 1

Achieving Your Ultimate You

MUCH OF LIFE IS BEYOND our control—our crazy bosses, our turbulent relationships, whether we get into a fender bender on the way home from the grocery store.

But there is one thing you can control: your weight.

Seriously—you really can. And this is coming from a certified personal trainer who whips actresses, models, and everyday women into shape (Joe) and a naturopathic physician who specializes in weight loss and maintains a thriving practice in New York City (Dr. Brooke).

> There is one thing you can control: your weight.

Together, we've crafted a totally unique program that will allow you to control certain processes within your body that impact your hunger, your cravings, how much body fat you carry, and where you carry it. Any woman can create the perfect version of herself. All you need are the right tools.

And we're here to give them to you: Our mission is to help you achieve your ultimate body.

What that means in the real world is totally up to you. It might mean fitting into your favorite jeans and seeing some nice definition in your arms when you wear a tank top, or it may be feeling good about your abs when you put on a bikini. Whatever the particulars, you can have a lean, strong physique and achieve peak fitness, vitality, and health.

There's an old saying that goes, "You can't control the wind, but you can set your sails." That's what the Ultimate You program does: It teaches you to adjust the sail—

why is there always another weight-loss book?

Here's the truth: We don't know all there is to know about weight loss, nutrition, or exercise. Also, the published scientific literature is often well behind practical application in Joe's gym and at Dr. Brooke's office.

But here's another reason there's always another weight-loss book: Often the programs don't work . . . at least for the long term. Most offer a quick fix for—rather than a solution to—the underlying issues of how women become overweight in the first place. Issues like hormones and digestion and behaviors like emotional eating are often ignored in favor of the rapid weight loss (notice we didn't say *fat* loss) and short-term promises that you'll be bikini ready or one-up an old rival at a high-school reunion.

What's worse is many "diets" are unhealthy. Quick-fix plans in particular tend to be low calorie, super low carb, and too low on veggies and whole, natural foods, or they tout the use of chemical sweeteners.

If the book does address hormones, it tends to focus on how one hormone in isolation causes weight gain, such as one of the "hormone of the month" diets out there, and single-minded focus tends to wreak havoc on the balance of other hormones.

If the book touts natural, whole foods, the plan tends to be too high in carbs (often as whole grains, which raise insulin) or miss the point entirely (i.e., Asian cultures are healthy and they eat soy, so drink a bunch of soy milk and you'll be healthy, too). Although plans that have you eat whole foods are a step up from those that allow processed foods, they are still far from perfect.

Our book factors in all of those things. Think of your hormones as a symphony: multiple instruments that need to work together to create a wonderful whole. If the tuba player decides to play her own tune, the overall effect is . . . unpleasant! Whole foods and healthy food-related behaviors can help you achieve a harmonious balance.

Our plan is plant-based, emphasizing real, whole foods (but not excess grains). It's focused on fiber, quality protein, healthy fats, and managed carbs rather than no carbs, and it doesn't sacrifice one hormone for another.

Our plan also addresses the beneficial nutrients in certain foods that not only promote weight loss but help manage hormones. For example, we use veggie fiber to keep your tummy satisfied and "super-fats" like conjugated linoleic acid (CLA), found in grass-fed beef, and omega-3 fatty acids, found in fish, to balance hormones and melt belly fat.

Our overall aim is to address the underlying issues of weight gain—to fix the problems, not the symptoms. We also want to teach women how their hormones influence fat gain and fat loss and how to manipulate them easily and naturally.

It all comes back to control—we want to put it back where it belongs: in your hands.

that is, to manipulate your hormones to encourage your body to burn fat and discourage it from storing fat. How?

You'll achieve this through **proper nutritional habits, smart exercise, managed stress,** and **better sleep.**

Here's how Ultimate You is different from every other book or program you've ever seen: This isn't a weight-loss plan. It's a *fat-loss* plan that uses a revolutionary concept—*metabolic disturbance*—to set in motion an almost magical fat-burning environment within your body. This environment switches on fat-burning hormones during your workout and creates a post-workout "afterburn" that burns calories hours after you leave the gym.

You've probably tried the old "move more, eat less" weight-loss advice, with little to show for it. It's not your fault. That paradigm might help you lose weight—for a little while, anyway—but it won't help you lose fat, which is what you want.

On the Ultimate You program, you'll eat better, move smarter, and lose body fat from all over. Joe gives you the workouts. Dr. Brooke's in charge of the nutrition and lifestyle program. Together, we offer a plan that can help you reach your ultimate best in size, shape, and health.

> On the Ultimate You program, you'll eat better, move smarter.

We've used these protocols to help our clients achieve the bodies they want. Funny thing is, many of them have told us that, along the way to achieving peak physical results, they became the people they always wanted to be. That's why we called our program Ultimate You: It introduces you to your best, healthiest, most vital self.

So prepare to take control, get lean, and meet your Ultimate You. (And do take the time to do the little visualization on page 9.)

But first, let us explain what you've probably been doing wrong and how to make it right.

TURNING METABOLIC CALM TO CHAOS

You can't achieve an Ultimate You body by sticking to the same low- to medium-intensity workout over and over again. First, you'll be bored to tears and will likely quit. Second, within as little as a few weeks, your body will adjust to those movements and that level of effort—and burn fewer calories.

Ultimate You workouts are based on the principle of metabolic disturbance, and they turn your body into a calorie-burning machine, which will ultimately lead to less body fat.

Your body is adaptive—it does what it must to survive and work at peak efficiency. You see this adaptive quality in action when you cut calories to lose weight.

If you drastically reduce calories, your body thinks it's starving. In response, to conserve fuel, it uses the paltry amount of calories it does get more efficiently. Result: Your metabolism slows.

The same dynamic applies when you run on a treadmill every day for 40 minutes or repeat the same strength-training routine for months on end—your body adjusts to that routine to conserve energy. Result: The same effort burns fewer calories.

The workouts you'll find in this book—which team total-body strength training with moderate- to high-intensity interval training—recruit the greatest amount of muscle fibers and trigger the greatest release of anabolic fat-burning hormones. Why is all this desirable? This is where the hormonal stuff comes in.

As you perform the workouts, you create a "metabolic storm" inside your body. That storm sets in motion a cascade of hormones that burn fat and maintain lean muscle tissue.

Metabolic disturbance also raises what exercise physiologists call EPOC, or excessive post-exercise oxygen consumption. You can call it workout afterburn.

Because these workouts create metabolic chaos, your body takes a long time to return to baseline (scientists call this *homeostasis*). Your body expends energy—calories—to return to homeostasis. The greater the disruption, the longer it takes to return to homeostasis. Result: You burn more calories after your workout.

It's the afterburn that counts.

That last point is critical, because the key to fat loss is not necessarily the calories you expend during an actual workout but the increased caloric expenditure that occurs over the 24- to 48-hour period following the workout. In other words, it's the afterburn that counts.

Light- to medium-intensity exercise—say, brisk walking on a treadmill—raises afterburn for mere minutes after you quit. The moderate- to high-intensity Ultimate You workouts, on the other hand, keep your metabolism revving for hours after your workout ends—even at rest.

THE HORMONE CONNECTION

Weight loss is all about metabolism—how quickly your body burns calories directly affects the number on the scale. That's what most people think, anyway.

Metabolism doesn't regulate body weight and calorie burn alone. Those two functions are a small part of your metabolism's primary mission: to keep you alive and breathing.

Plus, your metabolism itself has a master: your hormones. This beautifully orchestrated system of chemical messengers can dramatically affect your shape and size. Hormones determine how much fat you carry. Hormones dictate where you carry it—around your belly (cortisol), from your midsection to bra line (insulin), on your hips and thighs (estrogen). Hormones control your sensation of satiety—that is, whether you feel pleasantly full or constantly hungry—as well as your cravings.

No doubt you've heard a lot about the impact of two hormones in particular—insulin and cortisol—on weight. Well, they do affect weight, but you can't look at hormones in a vacuum; they work together, in concert. Indeed, experts speak of the body's hormonal symphony—just like the instruments in an orchestra, the combined effect of hormones is more important than the effect of any one hormone. So you can't blame just insulin or just cortisol for your extra pounds.

Besides insulin and cortisol, other hormones influence fat loss (testosterone and growth hormone, which we call your lean hormones), appetite (cholecystokinin, or CCK, ghrelin, neuropeptide Y, and leptin), and fat storage (estrogen and insulin).

And guess what? When one is unbalanced, it's only a matter of time until others become unbalanced, which isn't good news. For example, your breast tissue doesn't care if you stick to 1,200 calories a day. But when it comes to PMS breast tenderness and breast cancer risk, it certainly does matter that your insulin levels are high and your estrogen balance is off. What we're trying to say is that while hormones affect your weight, they have a profound effect on your health.

We'll examine hormones in detail later on. For now, you need to know just two things.

1. To have a healthy metabolism, *all* your hormones must be in balance.
2. Poor diet, high stress levels, working out incorrectly, and toxins in the environment can send hormones precariously out of whack, which can cause weight gain and other health issues.

what is a naturopathic doctor?

You might be wondering: Is Dr. Brooke a real doctor?

Yes, she is. As a licensed naturopathic doctor (ND), she attended a 4-year post-graduate naturopathic medical school, completed internships and residencies, and passed two levels of rigorous board exams.

A licensed ND is a primary-care doctor—like your family physician or GP—who supports your body's healing by utilizing six key principles.

1. Choose treatments that aim to do no harm.
2. Be a teacher and guide to the patient (*docere*).
3. Support the body's natural ability to self-heal (*vis medicatrix naturae*).
4. Identify and treat the cause of the illness rather than its symptoms.
5. Aid in prevention (the idea is to become more healthy rather than less ill).
6. Treat the whole person, not merely any one symptom or disease.

Hippocrates, sometimes considered the first physician in the naturopathic tradition, operated on the premise that "nature is healer of all diseases." Honoring this tradition, licensed NDs rely heavily on natural and nutritional therapies. However, they are also skilled in conventional diagnoses and treatment, meaning that your health is always in medically trained hands. Many NDs use conventional therapies, like prescription medications, alongside more alternative, natural treatments.

Regulation for NDs varies from state to state. If you seek the care of an ND, ensure the practitioner is licensed, and inquire where he or she received his or her degree—it should be from one of the institutions below, which are the only accredited naturopathic medical schools in North America.

- Bastyr University
- University of Bridgeport College of Naturopathic Medicine
- National College of Natural Medicine
- Southwest College of Naturopathic Medicine
- Boucher Institute of Naturopathic Medicine
- Canadian College of Naturopathic Medicine
- National University of Health Sciences

To find a licensed ND in your area, log on to the American Association of Naturopathic Physicians' Web site at www.naturopathic.org.

There is a silver lining, though: While hormone imbalance can wreak havoc with your ability to lose fat, metabolic disturbance, coupled with a healthy lifestyle and the right nutrition, can treat it and even prevent it.

HOW THE PROGRAM WORKS

The Ultimate You program is broken into four 4-week phases that encompass workouts and a nutrition/lifestyle program. Four weeks is how long it takes, on average, for the body to get used to a fitness routine. Four phases challenge your body progressively with more demands.

Like the workouts, the nutrition and lifestyle plans change from phase to phase, with each phase building upon the last. While the workouts are designed to create a metabolic disturbance, the nutrition and lifestyle changes are designed to restore balance to your body so that you get the most out of the workouts. Throughout the program, you'll correct the metabolic or hormonal issues that are affecting your health and your physique.

The nutrition and lifestyle plans have two tracks: one kinder, gentler track and one that's more strict for faster and more dramatic results. Regardless of which track you choose (and you may oscillate between the two), you'll lose body fat and improve your health.

The Ultimate You Workouts

Here's a brief description of the phases.

- **Phase 1—Preparation:** In this launch phase, you will focus on base conditioning and increasing muscular endurance and core strength.

- **Phase 2—Accumulation:** In this phase, you'll step up the intensity of your resistance training workouts, which will help increase your lean muscle mass and reduce

gym phobic?

You may be saying to yourself now, *Time to put the book down. I don't do gyms.* Give it a chance: The first few phases will build your confidence and stamina, and by the time you reach the phase that requires gym workouts, you'll have everything you need to feel at ease working out in public! When that time arrives, we'll give you some pointers about making smart choices when it comes to gyms and trainers.

If you decide to join a gym, take advantage of the less accessible recovery protocols of the Ultimate You program, which are just as important as the actual workouts. Yes, you can draw yourself a nice bath at home, but your gym may have a fuller spectrum of resources like a sauna, a stretching area, or spa/massage services. All good reasons to join!

body fat. In addition, you'll ramp up the intensity of your training with anaerobic intervals.

- **Phase 3—Intensification:** As you continue to increase your lean muscle and lose body fat, the intensity of your anaerobic intervals will further escalate. You'll also be introduced to circuit training.

- **Phase 4—Ultimate You:** You'll begin to perform total-body resistance-training circuits while focusing on increasing the density of the workouts, doing more work in a shorter amount of time. You'll push the intensity even more. Of course, you'll continue to build lean muscle and burn fat.

Although you can perform Phases 1 through 3 either at home or in the gym, we encourage you to join a gym—Joe has found that his clients encounter fewer distractions at a gym, which means they see results sooner. You'll need to do Phase 4 in a gym—the phase requires the use of several different cardio machines and special strength-training equipment that are not practical for home workouts.

The Ultimate You Nutrition/Lifestyle Plan

No more counting grams of *anything*. This high-fiber, high-protein plan is built on a scientific fact: By managing what you eat and when you eat it, you can create a hormonal environment that burns fat, discourages fat storage, promotes leanness, builds calorie-burning muscle, and manages satiety and cravings.

> By managing what you eat and when you eat it, you can create a hormonal environment that burns fat, discourages fat storage, promotes leanness, builds calorie-burning muscle, and manages satiety and cravings.

And it's so simple (and tasty) to eat this way. Simply choose your foods from our "Optimal" and "Allowable" lists (see pages 75 to 84).

Optimal foods are plant fibers (veggies and fruits), smart carbs from plant sources (i.e., high-fiber fruits and root veggies like yams and sweet potatoes), and lean proteins that are organic and hormone free. These foods create the optimal hormonal environment in which to burn fat; they also promote good health and digestion and keep your tummy satisfied. Other Optimal foods include healthy fats such as nuts, avocado, coconut, and olive oil. By the way, you'll be eating lots of green veggies, even with breakfast—they offer the fiber you want without the

self, meet your ultimate you

Before you begin the program, we want you to get acquainted with your Ultimate You. This is the version of yourself you might secretly wish for: The *you* that can fit into a particular size of jeans. The *you* that feels good when she walks down the street. The *you* that doesn't binge on a bag of potato chips and feel terrible afterward!

Or your Ultimate You may have nothing to do with dress size or food. You may have other dreams and goals in mind. Don't hold back: This is just your imagination here, so there's no reason you can't let loose and be a little crazy in your goal setting. Want to scale a mountain? In order to achieve great things, you have to think great thoughts!

Or maybe you've been so overwhelmed by life that you haven't been able to even take the time to envision that best version of yourself! But here's your opportunity to imagine: What does she look like? And just as important, how does she feel? What does she do?

Close your eyes and let her take shape in your mind (first impressions count). Then write down what you see. These questions can help get you started.

■ What is your Ultimate You wearing?

■ What is she doing? Lifting weights at the gym? Strolling down the beach in a two-piece swimsuit? Packing up a closet full of clothes that are now too big? Glancing in a full-length mirror, smiling at her new fit body? Perhaps she's doing something she's always wanted to do—taking a belly-dancing class, running for town council—but never had the self-confidence to try.

■ If you were to peek at the tag on her jeans or dress, what would the size be?

■ If you were to describe your Ultimate You in three words, what would they be?

MY ULTIMATE OUTFIT:

_____

_____

_____

_____

MY ULTIMATE ACTIVITIES:

_____

_____

_____

_____

MY ULTIMATE DRESS SIZE:

_____

_____

THE ULTIMATE ME IN THREE WORDS:

_____

_____

_____

starchy carbs you don't, and they are packed with healthy antioxidants and plant nutrients to boot.

Allowable foods include low-fat dairy and a few other high-fiber carbs like hemp or sprouted-grain bread, steel-cut oats, and high-fiber crackers. But these grain-based products are secondary to the "smarter" plant foods like root veggies and fruit. Still, Allowable foods expand your meal options and give you more flexibility when you dine out or when you need a break, while still keeping you on plan.

As previously mentioned, you won't count calories, carbs, or fat grams. That said, the plan provides guidelines for protein and carbohydrate servings that you can use until you learn to "read" your body and know which foods keep you leaner/losing fat and which don't. Every body is different, and the Ultimate You program will definitely give you the guidelines you need to get lean and stay that way, but it'll require you to pay attention to how your body is responding to what you put in it. Don't worry—we'll guide you through every step of the way.

> You'll be working hard, so once a week, reward yourself with a splurge meal.

You'll be working hard, so once a week, reward yourself with a splurge meal. Feel free to enjoy a higher-calorie, higher-carb indulgence, and maybe even have a glass of wine. Indulging will actually reset some key hormones by sending the message to your body that you aren't in starvation mode, which keeps your metabolism cranked up and your body burning fat.

HOW TO USE THIS BOOK

You're setting out on an adventure to find your Ultimate You—and every journey needs a map! Read on to find out where you're going and how you'll get there.

Chapters 2 and 3 are primers for strength-training and energy system training (EST) workouts. Whether you'll train at home or at the gym, you'll get all the information you need to hit the ground running on Day 1 of Phase 1, including a list of the equipment you'll need and tips that will help you maximize your workouts.

Although you'll train hard, your muscles need downtime to recover. In Chapter 4, you'll learn why recovery and regeneration, or R&R, is as important as training and how to give your body the rest it needs to grow lean and strong. You'll also get the recipe for the Ultimate You Recovery Shake, which you'll sip after each strength-training session throughout the program.

Don't know much about hormones? You will after you finish Chapter 5. You'll discover how they regulate your shape, size, weight, and appetite and how to manipulate them to rev up your body's ability to burn fat.

How does a high-fiber diet promote leanness? Why does eating fat help you lose fat? Chapter 6, "Fueling the Ultimate You," gives you answers, lays out the plan's nutritional guidelines, and presents the Optimal and Allowable foods lists.

Before you jump into the program, you'll need to shop for the food and supplements you'll need, give your kitchen an Ultimate You makeover, and learn to handle situations that can derail your program, like cravings and eating out. You'll find a step-by-step countdown in Chapter 7, "Preparing for the Ultimate You."

Chapters 8 to 11 are the core of the book: the four phases. Each chapter lays out that phase's workout and nutrition and lifestyle recommendations, with an emphasis on hormonal manipulation.

the ultimate story

Dr. Brooke and I met in late 2008, after Tim, the director of personal training at Peak Performance, my gym, told me about a client who was working with a naturopathic doctor and having tremendous success.

"The doctor would be interested in doing a couple of lectures," he added. Since I am always looking for cutting-edge health practitioners to educate my trainers, I called to invite her to speak.

Dr. Brooke presented the basics of nutrition alongside more advanced ideas: why it's important to eat high-quality protein, the effect of hormones on weight, and how estrogen dominance affects health and weight.

I thought, *Wow! We're on the same page.* I knew I really liked her when, in the Q&A session afterward, one of my trainers asked about portion control.

"How do you get your clients to eat less?" the trainer asked.

"It's not about eating less," Dr. Brooke said. "It's about eating better. No one gets fat eating grilled salmon and salad." She explained that whole, natural foods encourage the release of hormones that burn fat and promote satiety. I was sold. A few weeks after we met, we decided to collaborate on this book.

—Joe Dowdell

Since the Ultimate You program is a way of life, you're never "done." Once you've completed Phase 4, you'll want to keep the leaner, healthier body you've worked so hard to achieve. Chapter 12, "What Now?" tells you how to maintain your gains. If you're not quite where you want to be, you'll find helpful advice (and some new tips) that will get you to your goal.

The Appendix contains even more tools to help you succeed, such as delicious meal ideas, a supplement schedule, and a training log to record your workouts and track your progress.

Here's the really good news: It won't take long to see progress. With each phase you complete, you'll reach a new level of physical and mental well-being. Your workouts will begin to invigorate rather than intimidate. You'll crave whole, natural foods instead of the toxic stuff that passes for food. As your percentage of body fat falls, your self-confidence will rise. And somewhere along the way, you'll catch sight of your reflection—maybe in the mirrored walls of the gym or as you pass a shop window—and there she'll be: your Ultimate You.

CHAPTER 2

Resistance Training

BELIEVE US, WE'VE HEARD EVERY excuse in the book when it comes to why women don't want to lift weights. Most of them boil down to this: "I don't want to get big." Well, forget everything you think you know.

Fear not—you won't bulk up like a man. In fact, most *men* can't bulk up the way they'd like to. Bottom line: Women have lower levels of testosterone, so it's virtually impossible for you to get huge without steroids or the genetic propensity to pile on muscle. Worry about climate change or your 401(k), but don't worry that if you lift heavy weights you will turn into Hulkette.

Resistance training—also known as strength training or simply lifting weights— refers to exercises that build muscle by harnessing an opposing force that muscles must work against. This resistance can come from your own body weight (such as pushups or chinups), free weights (such as dumbbells and barbells), elasticized bands or tubing, or specialized machines at the gym.

WHY WEIGHTS?

The effectiveness of strength training boils down to what is called the *progressive overload* of skeletal muscles. In other words, it pushes those muscles harder than they're used to working, in a systematic and gradual manner.

Strength training (any voluntary movement you make, actually) is made possible

the side benefits of pumping iron

Strength training builds more than a sleeker, fitter physique: It builds good health. Research shows that people who lift weights a few times a week accrue many benefits.

■ **Stronger bones:** As a weight-bearing exercise, lifting weights improves the strength of your bones, which lowers your risk of osteoporosis later on.

■ **Weight loss and weight control:** Want to rev your metabolism by as much as 15 percent? Hit the weights, ladies. The more muscle you have, the higher and hotter your metabolism burns. That's because muscle is active tissue that consumes calories (body fat, on the other hand, uses very few). Metabolism can stay elevated for up to 24 hours post-workout, even longer than after a long session on the treadmill. This means you'll burn more calories more quickly, even as you sleep.

■ **Reduced risk of injury:** Build muscle and you protect your joints. Strength training also helps you maintain flexibility and balance and remain independent as you age.

■ **Increased stamina:** As you grow stronger, you won't fatigue as easily.

■ **Improved sense of well-being:** When you lift weights, your mood brightens, your mind sharpens, and your self-confidence soars. In fact, research has found that strength training provides similar improvements in depression to antidepressant medications.

■ **Better-quality sleep:** People who lift weights regularly tend to fall asleep more quickly, sleep more deeply, awaken less often, and sleep longer, research shows.

■ **Improved current and future health:** If you need to improve your blood pressure or blood cholesterol levels—or if you have pre-diabetes or diabetes and need to watch your blood sugar—strength training can help, studies have found.

by the body's 600-odd skeletal muscles, which are fused to bone. Every time you lift, those muscle fibers suffer microscopic tears (which sounds worse than it is). The body responds to these tears by making more and bigger proteins, which translates into bigger muscles. Because the muscles being worked tug on underlying bone, resistance training strengthens your bones, too.

While the process of tearing down and rebuilding muscle is complex, here's the basic process in a nutshell. When you lift, damaged muscle tissues release signaling factors—substances that attract immune cells to the damaged site. The immune cells trigger inflammation. This process is designed to remove damaged tissue from around the torn fibers. (If you've overdone it, this inflammation can leave you incredibly sore. If you've lifted smart, however, you'll just feel a pleasant tightness.)

The immune cells release substances that stimulate the production of satellite cells. Stimulated by hormones and other anabolic chemicals, these satellite cells then merge with the muscle cells as part of the repair process. At the end of the process, the muscle tear is repaired. But the muscle itself isn't quite the same one you had before because it's gained additional and larger cells. Not only is the muscle stronger, it's denser— muscle takes up less space than body fat.

Strength training does more than give you a bikini-ready body, though. It also increases the muscular strength and endurance you depend on as you perform your everyday activities, from painting a room to carrying groceries from your car to your kitchen. Your golf or tennis game stands to improve, too, and you'll find that you can work in your garden or keep up with your kids for longer periods without pooping out. You look better, but you feel better, too, mentally as well as physically.

THE ULTIMATE YOU DIFFERENCE

There are several things that make our approach to strength training different from other programs you may have tried.

- **Our workout is designed to impact the hormonal system.** Strength training impacts the muscular and nervous systems, but most programs don't address the hormonal system—and as you now know, hormones like insulin, growth hormone, and cortisol can dramatically impact body composition. That's why you need to use our nutrition program and recovery-and-regeneration techniques (Chapter 4) in tandem with the strength program. If you don't take advantage of these critical factors, you will limit your gains.

- **Each phase systematically and strategically progresses.** As we mentioned, the Ultimate You program emphasizes the progressive-overload approach to resistance training. That is, you'll increase the stress (i.e., demands) on your body systematically and gradually, from workout to workout and phase to phase. The result: Your body is continually forced to adapt to ever-increasing challenges, which promotes that all-important metabolic disturbance.

  We'll ramp up the training effect in several ways. First, you will progress

The heavier you lift, the leaner you'll get.

from simple movements to more challenging ones. Second, you will increase the *intensity* of your workouts—that is, you will train progressively harder in each phase. Third, you will increase the *density* of those workouts, so you do more work in less time. Increasing intensity and density, in particular, optimizes fat loss.

Of course, you will progress in a safe but effective way. It does you no good to work out too hard too fast, only to suffer pain or injury. This is a lifelong program, after all.

- **Our program emphasizes full-body routines.** Each session works your whole body, as opposed to split routines, which work one particular body part (i.e., biceps, triceps, or glutes). And for our money, full-body routines are the way to go. First, they're time efficient. More important, though, compared with split routines, full-body routines allow for greater energy expenditure, greater increase in metabolism, and greater hormonal response per workout. All of those benefits add up to more fat loss.

- **Our program features two phases to the warmups that properly prepare your body to train.** Our workouts change frequently. That means the warmups need to change, too. Walking on the treadmill for 5 minutes or pedaling a stationary bike doesn't cut it. A general warmup like that won't work the joints you'll be using for specific movements or cue the nervous system for the movements you will do. Our two-step warmup process—called *dynamic warmup* and *activation drills*—is tailored to the strength-training exercises in that particular phase.

Dynamic warmups prime your joints and muscles for specific exercises. For example, when you perform squats, your dynamic warmup will prepare your ankles, knees, and

---

the heavier you lift, the leaner you'll get

Many women refuse to lift heavy weights—or lift weights at all—for fear they will get bulky. If you have this fear, please lay it to rest right now.

Unless they use steroids, women cannot put on muscle the way men do when they lift heavy. It's physically impossible—women simply do not have enough testosterone.

When you start to lift weights, you may build up a bit of muscle under your layer of body fat, so you feel bulkier. But if you eat clean and do your EST (more about what this means in Chapter 3), you will lose that puffy look and gain muscle that looks lean and sexy, not bulky.

Another thing—when you first start to lift weights, your muscles will need to store more sugar as glycogen. This process can cause you to gain a few pounds of water, which is typically gone within a week or two.

burn more fat or fizzle out?
the pre-workout nutrition question

Pre-workout nutrition is a hotly debated topic in the fitness industry. "Work out fasted and on empty to burn more fat," some say. Others retort, "No, no! Fuel up to avoid crashing during a session." Taking our collective years of experience and the current science, the Ultimate You pre-workout advice is somewhere in the middle.

Across the board, low-intensity exercise (like the long walks we recommend later in the book) appears to burn more fat and not create exaggerated hormone responses if done fasting and first thing in the morning. Beyond that, it's a little tricky. If you are following your nutrition plan every day and eating regularly, you'll likely have plenty of stamina for your workouts regardless of how much attention you pay to pre-workout fueling. However, use these guidelines to get the most out of your sessions.

For morning EST sessions:

■ If you feel energized upon waking, go ahead and hit the gym on empty. This will raise your cortisol maximally during your session; research shows this is a powerful stimulant for fat burning.

■ If you wake up feeling nauseated or unrested, utilize a quickly absorbed protein shake about 1 hour prior to your session. Try this recipe: Mix ½ cup Ultimate Whey (Hardware) with ½ cup coconut water or regular water; blend with ice if desired. Avoid high-carb meals like oatmeal, fruit, or even yogurt to avoid spiking insulin, which will hinder fat burning.

For morning strength-training sessions:

■ Use the above protein shake recipe 60 to 90 minutes prior to your strength-training session.

For afternoon/evening EST or strength-training sessions:

■ Plan your meal schedule so that you have any bigger meal (i.e., breakfast or lunch) at least 2 hours before your session or have a snack at least 90 minutes prior.

These guidelines will help you read your body and fuel according to what feels best to you. Having your cortisol rhythms evaluated by a health-care provider can allow you to further fine-tune your regimen.

hip joints for that particular exercise. Activation drills "wake up" muscles that are typically underutilized or inherently weak. They turn on the light so that you perform the rest of your workout in a bright room.

To optimize the *anabolic* (muscle building) response to training and minimize the *catabolic* (muscle breakdown) response, our workouts are designed to take under an hour, including the warmup and cooldown. A 45-minute workout is optimal—that's when testosterone levels start to drop and cortisol levels increase dramatically.

These workouts also aim to trigger an acute growth hormone response, which helps increase lean muscle mass and decrease body fat. To trigger this response, you'll team moderate to heavy resistance with a brief rest period (30 to 60 seconds per exercise) between each set and/or circuit of exercises. (Note that the rest period can be as long as 2 minutes after the Phase 4 total-body circuits.)

HOME OR GYM?

Many women exercise at home and love it. There are solid reasons to work out at home—perhaps finances are an issue, or you want to lose a few pounds before you "go public" in a gym environment. And once you have the right equipment, working out at home is free, convenient, and private.

We've designed this program so that you can complete the first three phases at home. That said, we recommend that you train in a gym if possible. There are several reasons for this.

First, a gym has more room and better equipment. You need a pretty sophisticated home setup to match a large gym environment. Second, it's been our experience that people are more motivated in a gym setting. They see other people training hard and step up their own workouts. There are also fewer distractions at a gym—no phone calls, children, or spouses—just you and the weights. Finally, trainers are usually available—and free—to provide advice.

So if you can swing it, join a gym—your body will reflect your investment. But don't just join a gym—join the *right* gym for *you*. Here are three "must-haves."

1. **A friendly vibe:** Before you join a gym, drop in a few times for a couple of scans of the room and ask yourself, *Do these people seem like the type of people I'd feel comfortable working out with?* If the answer is no, keep looking.

2. **Experienced, credentialed trainers:** Before you trust a trainer with your body, check his or her qualifications. You want to hear that he or she is certified by the

American College of Sports Medicine, American Council on Exercise, National Strength and Conditioning Association, or National Academy of Sports Medicine. Also, ask if there are trainers stationed on the gym floor when they are not working with clients.

3. **Clean, pleasant surroundings:** Your mental well-being is as important as your physical well-being, and if you're working out in a dark, dreary gym just to save la few bucks, you probably won't want to go there too often. Make sure the gym you join is one part of each day that you truly look forward to.

WHAT YOU NEED TO SUCCEED

Strength training isn't rocket science, but there are definitely "rules of the road" that will help you train safely and effectively. To get the most out of our program, follow these tips.

- **When possible, use body weight, free weights, and cable-based exercises.** The Ultimate You program emphasizes exercises that use the weight of your own body, dumbbells, or cables over machine-based exercises. Not only are these exercises more efficient for overall fitness and fat loss, they also engage more muscle groups during any given movement pattern. This activation of muscles as stabilizers has a greater transfer to activities of daily living and sport.

- **Keep moving.** You'll lose more fat—and get in and out of the gym faster— if you use the multiple-station approach of exercise sequencing. For example, perform 1 set of 1 exercise (such as squats); rest 60 seconds; perform 1 set of the next exercise (such as chinups); rest 60 seconds. By pairing these 2 exercises, you let your lower body recover while your upper body is working and vice versa.

- **Log your workouts.** You *must* use the training log to keep track of the resistance chosen for each exercise and the number of reps performed with that resistance during each set. In fact, we recommend recording the weight selected and the number of reps performed after each set. We find that ensures that you have an accurate record of the workout, and it also keeps you focused on the

home-gym essentials

Dumbbells: There are two basic types: fixed-weight and adjustable. Fixed-weight dumbbells are commonly found in gyms. They're effective, but in the home setting, you would need several pairs of different weights so you could gradually increase the amount you lift over the course of your training phases.

Adjustable dumbbells allow you to add or remove individual weight plates. We recommend the PowerBlock SportBlock, which lets you lift from 3 to 24 pounds. You can safely adjust the weight in seconds, and it's great if you're cramped for space. They're relatively inexpensive, too.

Adjustable weight bench: You don't need to spend hundreds of dollars. Look for a well-made, sturdy bench that has good padding.

Exercise mat: This is a must-have. A mat will cushion you from the hard floor when you perform your warmup and cooldown routines, as well as floor exercises.

Swiss ball: A Swiss ball—or stability ball—helps strengthen nearly every muscle in your body as it improves balance, coordination, and posture. Stability balls come in various sizes, based on height. Use this guide to choose the ball that's right for you.

Your Height	Proper Sizing
4'6" to 5'0"	45 cm (18") ball
5'1" to 5'7"	55 cm (22") ball
5'8" to 6'2"	65 cm (26") ball

Exercise bands: Diversity is the key to creating metabolic disturbance. These flexible, stretchable bands with handles on the ends provide a different type of resistance than dumbbells. A bonus: They're portable, so you can easily take them along when you travel. Exercise bands come in several color-coded levels of difficulty. Purchase them in two or three different levels so you can ramp up the challenge as your strength increases.

Jump rope: Most ropes come in 9- or 10-foot lengths. To determine the correct length for you, step one foot in the middle of the rope; the handles should reach your armpits.

Foam roller or The Stick: As you'll learn, allowing your muscles to recover is just as important as training them hard. These products are used post-workout to accelerate recovery of the muscles you've just trained. The main difference between the two: You place a foam roller on the floor and roll your body on it; you hold The Stick in your hands and roll it up and down your muscles.

Weighted vest (optional): Xvest makes a great weighted vest. But if you want the challenge without the cost, wear a backpack that contains 5 or 10 pounds of books—ideally, textbook-size.

Timer or stopwatch: You will need a device to keep track of time so you can adhere to prescribed rest periods.

training session. You'll find the log on page 258 or you can download a free copy at www.bodybyhardware.com.

- **Follow each phase's training schedule to the letter.** No matter how much you want sleek upper arms or nicely defined shoulders, do not train your triceps or shoulders 2 or more days in a row. You'll accomplish nothing but make those muscles sore or prone to injury.

- **Lift the right amount of weight. Make sure that the last repetition you can perform with proper form falls within the prescribed rep bracket.** (A repetition, or rep, is 1 repetition of a particular exercise. A set is a group of reps.) Once you can complete the maximum number of reps (i.e., 12 reps in a 10- to 12-repetition bracket) for the maximum number of sets (i.e., 3 sets), increase the resistance only slightly for the next workout. This increase should allow you to perform at least the minimum number of reps for all sets of the exercise. As a general rule of thumb and to make things relatively simple for you, try to increase the resistance by 5 to 10 pounds for lower-body dominant movements, such as the deadlift, and increase the resistance by 2½ to 5 pounds for upper-body movements, such as the dumbbell bench press.

- **How you lift is as important as how much you lift.** The goal is to stress your muscles and joints in a positive manner. Lift smoothly and with control. Don't use momentum to jerk the weight up. If you're using a machine, don't let the weight stack slam the bottom plate when you lower the weight.

- **Breathe naturally throughout the set.** Exhale during the most strenuous phase of the movement—usually, as you lift the weight. Inhale during the less strenuous phase—usually, as you return to the starting position. Never hold your breath as you train with weights, which could cause a potentially dangerous rise in blood pressure.

- **Get good-quality sleep.** Sleep helps your muscles recover. You can't train at your best on less than 7 to 8 hours.

- **If you need help, find it.** If you feel lost in the gym, find a trainer—he or she will be glad to answer any questions you might have. Don't hesitate to take this book with you, either. Working from the book will ensure that you perform the exercises correctly. If you're working out at home and find yourself at sea, log on to our Web site: www.bodybyhardware.com.

CHAPTER 3

Energy System Training (EST)

AS ITS NAME IMPLIES, "CARDIO" conditions the cardiovascular system. It also utilizes your lean muscle mass to burn calories, which can help you lose those extra pounds.

If you're like most women, however, you tend to focus on how many calories your workout generates. And trust us: All too often, that "calories burned" indicator on cardio machines is off the mark.

With energy system training (EST), you'll focus not on the number of calories your body expends during your actual workout but on how many it burns *over a 24-hour cycle*. Forget about "burning fat" during your workout, too. Your goal is to deplete your glycogen stores and utilize the carbs you've consumed. After your workout, your body will replenish those stores by breaking down fat.

Here's one of the best things about EST: It doesn't last long. Your longest session will take all of 28 minutes, including your warmup and cooldown. That's a welcome change if you typically spend 45 to 60 minutes grinding it out on a cardio machine.

Before you can understand how EST works, you need to learn a few basic facts about cardiovascular exercise. One of the most important is that there are different types of cardio, and some get you lean better than others.

ALL CARDIO IS NOT CREATED EQUAL

If you're like most people, if you do cardio at all, you slog your way through it. You hop on a machine and walk, pedal, or climb for 45 minutes at a relatively easy pace.

In other words, you're doing what exercise geeks like us call low-intensity steady-state cardiovascular exercise. And we'd be willing to bet you dread it.

To add insult to injury, this kind of "hamster-wheel cardio" doesn't burn many calories during the actual workout. Nor does this slow-and-steady effort elevate your metabolism the rest of the day.

the HIIT advantage: aerobic and anaerobic cardio

To get lean, you need to burn calories both during and after your workout. To get that continuous burn, you need to perform cardiovascular exercise that's predominantly anaerobic in nature. The two methods of cardio utilize different metabolic processes and accomplish different goals. The main difference between them is whether they require the presence of oxygen to generate energy.

When you walk, jog, cycle, or swim at a low to moderate intensity, you are performing aerobic exercise (*aerobic* means "with oxygen"). They are repetitive activities that work your heart and lungs, training them to better deliver oxygen to your working muscles. Aerobic exercise can make you breathless, but you can sustain it for prolonged periods. During aerobic exercise, your body uses oxygen to burn both carbohydrates and fats to produce energy. We prefer this type of energy system training on recovery days. In addition, if you're peri- or postmenopausal, adding in a few extra low-intensity walks each week will help you burn additional calories without sacrificing your lean muscle mass or negatively impacting your cortisol levels.

With anaerobic exercise, your working muscles' need for oxygen exceeds the available supply. Because its intensity is very high—think sprinting or lifting heavy weights—you can perform it only in short bursts. This type of exercise burns only carbohydrates to produce energy.

Anaerobic exercise doesn't burn as many calories as an equivalent amount of aerobic exercise; however, short-burst, intense anaerobic work is critically important for weight loss. Here's why.

- **It raises resting metabolism.** This means you extend your calorie burn for hours after your workout. You'll also burn more calories throughout the day, even at rest.

- **It causes the increase in blood lactate levels.** This increase in turn signals your body to release growth hormone. As you now know, growth hormone signals the body to release fatty acids into the bloodstream, where they are burned off.

- **It encourages the development of lean muscle mass.** Anaerobic exercise creates a favorable hormonal environment because it increases testosterone, which helps increase lean muscle mass.

But we've got good news: You're about to get off that hamster wheel. In fact, with our method, you cut your cardio time by more than half. In the process, you'll stimulate fat-burning post-workout, boost your stamina and endurance, and rev up your resting metabolism so you burn more calories throughout the day, even at rest.

What's our method? It's called *high-intensity interval training*—or *HIIT* for short. And it's simple. In this method of cardiovascular exercise, you alternate periods of higher-intensity work with periods of lower-intensity recovery. When you increase intensity, you can perform the same amount of *total work* as in that hamster-wheel cardio—but in a fraction of the time.

> In the process, you'll stimulate fat-burning post-workout, boost your stamina and endurance, and rev up your resting metabolism so you burn more calories throughout the day, even at rest.

While this method is advanced—it's used by elite athletes, fitness enthusiasts, and serious recreational runners—HIIT can be modified for beginners as well, provided they're free of health problems.

Let us spell out just some of the ways HIIT can help you get lean, fit, and healthy.

- You'll burn more calories in less time.

- You'll improve your cardiovascular endurance.

- You'll increase your lean muscle mass and reduce muscle catabolism.

- You'll shake up your cardio routine and challenge yourself.

- Your body will adapt to high-energy demands and, in the process, develop a more efficient fuel-delivery and waste-removal process.

There's yet another benefit. Because you alternate between periods of steady-state and high-intensity exercise, HIIT trains both slow- and fast-twitch muscle fibers, which will improve your overall fitness and performance levels.

THE ULTIMATE YOU DIFFERENCE

So what's a typical EST session like? Well, it's not too difficult at first. In Phase 1, you'll perform aerobic intervals. You'll push yourself but only a little. Believe us, you'll be able to handle it.

In Phases 2 through 4, your training gets more challenging. Be prepared: You will reach a point where you can't get enough oxygen to your working muscles to continue that level of effort. You might struggle for breath; your lungs or working muscles might burn.

Although that sounds bad, it isn't. Because HIIT challenges the body much more than the typical one-speed workout, it creates a major metabolic disturbance in your body, and that's what you want. You want to make sure that your body doesn't recover as quickly as it does from steady-state cardio, so it will burn more calories post-workout. This process, called excess post-exercise oxygen consumption (EPOC), is what revs up your metabolic rate.

If you're looking to lose fat, this "afterburn" will be of tremendous benefit. In a small but encouraging 2007 study, researchers from Canada had 8 young women complete 7 interval workouts, and whole-body fat oxidation among the interval-trained group increased 36 percent after performing HIIT, compared with low-intensity or moderate-intensity training. Better yet, these improvements were consistent regardless of the women's fitness level before they began HIIT.

> So how intense
> is intense? That
> depends on you.

So how intense is intense? That depends on you. Exercise too hard and your body won't be able to recover between sessions, and you'll burn out. On the other hand, if you don't exercise hard enough, you won't get the results you want. To reach your goal, it's important that you exercise at the correct intensity level for *you*.

To measure how hard your body is working, you will use several charts (see pages 28 to 29). The first chart estimates *rate of perceived exertion* (RPE). This subjective measure of physical effort is based on the sensations you experience during physical activity, such as faster breathing, sweating, and muscle fatigue.

A more objective and scientific approach to measuring exercise intensity, *target heart-rate training* allows you to measure intensity independently based solely on your heart rate. To keep things simple, you'll use five "zones," or training intensities, which you match to your RPE.

Remember to match the intensity of your workout effort to your fitness level. Take more recovery time if you need it, but experiment with raising intensity according to those charts. As your fitness improves, you're likely to find that you can work harder than you ever thought.

THE TYPICAL EST WORKOUT

Interval training burns fat, builds endurance, and helps maintain lean body mass. It also allows you to complete your workouts in a shorter period of time. Here's what you can expect.

- **WARMUP: 3 MINUTES**

  An EST session always begins with a 3-minute warmup. Don't skip it— warming up is important. It gradually raises your heart rate, sends blood to your working muscles, and ramps up your respiration. As a bonus, recent research suggests that warming up raises core body temperature and increases the activity of fat-burning enzymes.

- **INTERVAL TRAINING: 18 TO 28 MINUTES**

  In a typical EST session, after your 3-minute warmup, you will increase your intensity until you reach the recommended zone. You will hold this pace for 30 to 60 seconds. Then slow down to your normal tempo for 60 to 180 seconds, depending on the intensity of your work interval. You will repeat this work/recovery cycle for the recommended number of repetitions.

- **COOLDOWN: 3 MINUTES**

  Each EST session ends with a 3-minute cooldown. Don't skip this, either. The cooldown prevents the dizziness that can result when blood pools in the large muscles of the legs after vigorous activity is suddenly stopped. It also helps remove the metabolic waste products that can build up in muscles. Recirculating that waste and pooled blood will leave you feeling less fatigued post-workout.

- **POST-WORKOUT FOAM ROLLING: 7 MINUTES (APPROXIMATELY)**

  After your cooldown, it's time to get on it—your foam roller, that is. The poor (wo)man's massage improves flexibility and joint range of motion and helps to eliminate that "tight" feeling of overworked muscles. This allows you to train harder and recover more quickly while reducing the risk of injury. For more on the benefits of foam rolling, see Chapter 4.

● POST-WORKOUT STATIC STRETCHING: 7 MINUTES (APPROXIMATELY)

Stretching after your EST sessions—or better yet, after your strength-training sessions, too—can help you to relax after intense workouts and bring your stress hormones back down, and can potentially help to decrease injuries. Despite traditional advice, it's best to static stretch after exercise rather than before, and stretching should always be done after foam rolling. For more on static stretching, see Chapter 4.

the ultimate you RPE and HR training zone charts

The most accurate way to determine your true heart-rate training zones would be to perform a submax treadmill test, using a sophisticated system that a well-equipped gym would have. That said, you can use the following less sophisticated, more user-friendly method:

1. Subtract your age from 220. (This gives your age-predicted maximum heart rate.)
2. Multiply that number by the bottom- and top-end percentages for each zone in the heart-rate training zone chart below. (For example, 220 – 30 = 190; 190 x 50% = 95; and 190 x 59% = 112.)
3. Use those numbers to set your heart rate for each zone for a simple and reasonably accurate measure of how hard you should be working.

Heart-Rate Training Zone	% of Age-Predicted
1	50 to 59%
2	60 to 69%
3	70 to 79%
4	80 to 89%
5	90 to 100%

If you decide not to use a heart-rate monitor, the scale of rate of perceived exertion (RPE) can be very useful in helping to determine your effort level.

RPE	Level of Exertion	Quality of Breathing
1	Extremely easy	Very relaxed
2	Very easy	Can carry on a conversation (easily)

ARE YOU IN THE ZONE?
A HEART-RATE MONITOR CAN TELL YOU

A key principle of HIIT is that you must raise your heart rate above what you would normally experience with light or moderate cardio. That's why we recommend using a heart-rate monitor while you perform EST. Using a heart-rate monitor takes all the guesswork out of your workouts. It's also fun and gives you immediate feedback on whether you're working hard enough to squeeze the most benefit from your EST sessions.

RPE	Level of Exertion	Quality of Breathing
3	Easy	Can carry on a conversation (labored)
4	Moderate	Talking becomes difficult
5	Somewhat hard	Breathing becomes heavy
6	Moderately hard	Deep breaths; conversation avoided
7	Hard	Deep, forceful inhalation/expiration
8	Very hard	Labored breathing; cannot talk
9	Very, very hard	Very labored breathing
10	Extremely hard	Gasping and struggling for air

The formula for determining your training zone is not an exact science, so team a heart-rate monitor with the RPE scale. Using both will give you the most accurate assessment of your intensity level.

Heart-Rate and RPE Training Zones

HR Zone	Name	RPE
1	Active recovery	1 to 2
2	Aerobic threshold (extensive endurance)	3 to 4
3	Tempo (intensive endurance/ light- to moderate-intensity intervals)	5 to 6
4	Lactate threshold (moderate- to high-intensity intervals)	7 to 8
5	Anaerobic capacity (very high-intensity intervals)	9 to 10

While many cardio machines at your gym have built-in heart-rate monitors that will allow you to gauge your percentage of maximum heart rate, stand-alone heart-rate monitors are generally more reliable. There are several brands out there. Good heart-rate monitors can be found at most sporting-goods stores and start at around $50. We recommend the Polar brand (www.polarusa.com).

CARDIO OPTIONS FOR THE ULTIMATE YOU

We've designed the EST programs with specific cardio training in mind. For example, in Phase 1, we recommend treadmill training. In Phase 2, we suggest cycling. Below you'll find the most common—and effective—EST options.

- **Running:** It burns a tremendous amount of calories, and you can do it outside or on a treadmill. Running outside on a track or on the grass is ideal, but a treadmill is also effective and an excellent option in bad weather. The challenge with performing intervals on a treadmill is that it takes a few seconds to adjust the speed.

  Caveat: If you're new to exercise and/or significantly overweight, running is probably not the best option to start with. Before you begin to run, you need to develop an appropriate level of joint strength and stability. Our strength-training program will help you do that.

- **Cycling:** It is an excellent option for EST, especially in the early stages, as it allows you to work at higher intensities without fear of incurring an injury due to joint instability. Indoor cycling, sometimes known as Spinning, is another wonderful option for EST. For more information, visit www.spinning.com.

- **VersaClimber:** If your gym has this piece of equipment, we highly recommend it. Because you'll use both your upper and lower extremities, you'll burn tons of calories. The VersaClimber is also low impact, which reduces your chances of injury.

- **Rowing machine:** The indoor rower, such as the one made by Concept2, is an excellent piece of cardiovascular equipment. Like the VersaClimber, it is a low-impact device that requires you to use both your upper and lower body simultaneously.

Rowing is excellent for intervals. There is a slight learning curve, but proper technique is easy to pick up and wonderfully outlined on the Concept 2 Web site at www.concept2.com.

- **Jump rope:** This is an effective and inexpensive way to perform intervals. In addition, since it is so portable, it's excellent for travel. There is a bit of a learning curve to getting good at skipping rope, but your technique will improve over time. (More on skipping rope on page 199.)

- **Body-weight exercises:** You can perform these anywhere. Some of our favorites are jumping jacks, mountain climbers, squat thrusts, and low-box lateral shuffles.

WHAT YOU NEED TO SUCCEED

- **Train at the right time.** Perform the EST workout on the days between strength-training workouts so that you will be able to get the most out of each type of training.

- **Match your heart-rate training zone with your RPE.** That's what the charts on pages 28 to 29 are for—please use them. Also, feel free to scale these numbers up or down, based on how you feel. For example, if a certain zone seems too easy or too hard, increase or reduce your heart rate by five beats and reevaluate.

- **Push through slight nausea . . .** If you feel slightly sick to your stomach during EST, don't panic. That nausea means that you're working hard enough to create a lot of metabolic waste. The creation of that waste signals your body to release spurts of growth hormone. You'll find out all about those benefits when we tell you about balancing your hormones in Chapter 5. For now, know that the benefits include fat loss and an increase in lean body mass.

- **. . . But use common sense.** Don't work so hard that you really do get sick. If you fear you'll actually lose your last meal, reduce your effort.

CHAPTER 4

Recovery and Regeneration

WHEN IT COMES TO TRAINING, *recovery and regeneration*—R&R—are the magic words. You're training hard—you've earned it. More important, to get lean, strong, and fit, your body *needs* it. Recovery is an essential part of training. If you want a stronger, leaner body, you need to give your muscles the chance to recover.

Muscles repair, rebuild, and strengthen when you rest, not when you train. When you work out, your body breaks down muscle and depletes its fluids and energy stores. R&R allows your body to replenish those stores and repair those damaged tissues. A muscle needs anywhere from 24 to 48 hours to repair and rebuild, and working it again too soon can lead to muscle breakdown instead of gain.

> If you want a stronger, leaner body, you need to give your muscles the chance to recover.

Another thing: If you don't take recovery time between workouts, you risk overtraining. Working out too hard, too often, can result in injury, slowing your progress even further.

By contrast, R&R allows you to train harder, so you get more out of your workouts. By the way, lifestyle also influences recovery time. Eat well, sleep well, manage stress—in other words, live a health-conscious, balanced life—and your muscles will recover more quickly.

This chapter covers some of the best R&R techniques. Many are simple and inexpensive or even free. If your time and finances permit, you can try some of the more specialized (and pricey) methods.

R&R TOOLS 1 THROUGH 3

These are key elements of the Ultimate You program. You should treat them like religion! Sleep soundly every night, and do your static stretches and foam rolling nearly every day as part of your recovery routine.

R&R Tool #1: Sleep

Sound, restful sleep is the cornerstone of recovery. Enough sleep boosts lean hormones—growth hormone and testosterone, specifically. Restful sleep also allows for normal leptin secretion, which helps manage hunger. As if those benefits weren't enough, good sleep also keeps cortisol from getting too high the next day.

> Sound, restful sleep is the cornerstone of recovery.

HOW IT HELPS: While we sleep, several important physical processes occur, which help facilitate muscle growth and repair.

- The greatest secretion of growth hormone occurs during our deepest sleep cycles (i.e., stages 3 and 4).

- The body's metabolic activity is at its lowest point; therefore, we have an excellent environment for tissue repair.

HOW MUCH/HOW OFTEN: Typically, the average person needs from 6 to 8 hours of sound sleep per night to function optimally.

HOW TO USE IT: If you want to sleep like a rock, do not train within 4 hours of going to bed. Why? Because if cortisol and adrenaline levels are high from your workout, they will outweigh your parasympathetic nervous system, which signals your body that you're ready for sleep. The key is to keep cortisol lower instead of relying on the parasympathetic to take over. It also helps to switch off your TV and computer 2 hours before you hit the hay.

DR. BROOKE SAYS: Because of its effect on cortisol rhythms, lack of sleep increases cravings for sugary and fatty foods the next day. Good-quality sleep will make it much easier to stay on plan. And they don't call it beauty sleep for nothing! Lack of sleep and a poor diet will speed up aging faster than anything else. The Ultimate You plan is better than any anti-aging night cream, so get your zzz's.

R&R Tool #2: Foam Rolling

A form of self-massage using an object that looks a little like a swimming-pool noodle, foam rolling improves the quality of your muscle tissue. Specifically, the technique "irons out" knots (also known as trigger points) in the muscles.

A knot in a muscle is much like a knot in a rubber band. The "knot" is tissue that is dense and fibrotic, rather than smooth and pliable. Stretching can't get these knots out. Again, using the rubber-band analogy, if you pull on (stretch) the knot, it just gets tighter. Foam rolling improves the *quality* of muscle tissue, while stretching *lengthens* it.

HOW IT HELPS: The technique serves several purposes: pain reduction; injury prevention; and, ultimately, performance enhancement.

If you have knots inside the bellies of the muscle tissue, you have to iron them out. When a muscle has an area of increased density, no matter how much you stretch it, you will only improve the length of the tissue on either side of this trigger point. You cannot stretch out a trigger point—in fact, stretching can make the trigger point worse. If you encounter an area of increased density, which is usually associated with a sensation of sensitivity and pain, you will need to roll back and forth over that area for a longer period of time. You can then elongate that muscle by means of dynamic or static stretching.

HOW MUCH/HOW OFTEN: Ideally, it'll be done before every strength-training workout and prior to your static-stretching series, but at the very least, do it immediately after your EST sessions.

HOW TO USE IT: You'll perform eight foam-rolling exercises. They begin on page 42.

DR. BROOKE SAYS: I've found no better way to prevent workout-related injuries than foam rolling, which has the added advantage of breaking up adhesions between the muscle and skin layers, lending skin an even appearance.

R&R Tool #3: Static Stretching

Possibly the most common recovery technique of all is stretching. You've heard of it, you've most likely even done it—and yet it's one of the most misunderstood techniques around. Common misconceptions about stretching are that it creates longer, leaner muscles; that it's solely responsible for flexibility; and that it should be done prior to exercise to help decrease the risk of injury. What stretching actually does is temporarily lengthen muscles and tendons (one factor in overall flexibility) and, if done post-workout, relieve muscular tension and trigger the parasympathetic nervous system to help you relax.

The method employed here is known as *static stretching,* and involves you stretching a muscle, or group of muscles, to the point where you feel tension and then briefly holding. While you may be used to stretching before exercise, new research shows that pre-workout static stretching can actually decrease strength and power output and may even increase the risk of injury. So this recovery technique should only be done post-workout.

HOW IT HELPS: Stretching will help relieve built-up muscular tension from your workouts and bring down the cortisol response from intense exercise by increasing the output of the opposing parasympathetic system—helping you to literally unwind. When done regularly post-workout, it will contribute to improved flexibility, decreased injuries, and better overall musculoskeletal health.

HOW MUCH/HOW OFTEN: Ideally, 2 or 3 times per week, after your EST sessions, but may be performed after every workout. It should always be preceded by the foam rolling sequence.

HOW TO USE IT: For each muscle or group of muscles you are stretching, move into the stretch to the point where you feel tension and hold for 10 seconds (15 seconds max), then release. Take a deep breath and gently move back into the stretch, slightly deeper than before, to the point of tension and hold again for 10 seconds. Repeat this once more and then move on to the next muscle group. Be careful not to overstretch, as it can be damaging to the muscle, and always perform static stretching after foam rolling.

DR. BROOKE SAYS: Certain types of exercises that employ a lot of stretching have fostered the notion that they create "long, lean muscles." There are a couple of holes in that theory. First, stretching creates only a temporary lengthening of the muscle. Tendon and muscle lengths are preset in each of us—they are as long as they need to be in order to move the bone or bones they are attached to. And second, when it comes to a "lean muscle" . . . well, ladies, that isn't accomplished with stretching alone. A lean muscle is a muscle with very little fat over it. Stick with your Ultimate You nutrition plan and follow the exercise program in this book, and you'll be seeing those lean muscles in no time.

R&R TOOLS 4 THROUGH 9

You do not need to perform these daily, but you should included these steps as often as possible to keep your body injury free and feeling great. Some, like Epsom salt

the recovery shake

In Chapter 6, you'll learn more about how to eat to maximize the benefits of your workout and make the most of recovery and regeneration. Part of R&R is replacing the nutrients utilized during intense exercise. After the workouts outlined in this book, you are hormonally set up to burn fat for hours. To ensure that you are burning just fat and not muscle, a Recovery Shake is key. Follow the recipe below and consume within 1 hour after resistance training.

1 scoop whey protein (Ultimate Whey by Hardware or Jay Robb brand whey)

½ cup frozen berries

1 cup* liquid; try any of the following combinations:

1 cup water

OR ½ cup water and ½ cup coconut water

OR ½ cup water and ½ cup unsweetened vanilla or chocolate almond milk

* If you like a thicker shake, use less liquid; try ½ to ¾ cup total.

1 teaspoon unsweetened organic cocoa powder (optional)

5 to 10 grams L-glutamine powder (optional)

Your workouts become more intense during Phases 2 through 4; thus, you'll have a greater cortisol (a.k.a. stress) response from them. This jolt of cortisol actually burns more fat during a workout, but you'll want to squelch it post-workout. Sounds tricky, but an easy way to bring cortisol down is to bring insulin up. To do this, add 1 teaspoon honey or ½ cup grape juice to the Recovery Shake.

If you are insulin resistant or have diabetes (more on this in Chapter 5), you will not use honey, fruit, or fruit juice in your Recovery Shake—instead, add 15 grams L-glutamine, 15 grams glycine, and 10 grams leucine.

baths, are inexpensive and easy to integrate into your daily routine. On the other hand, tools like massage require a bit more planning but are well worth the time and expense! Aim to include one or two of these additional tools per week.

R&R Tool #4: Epsom Salt Baths

Draw a hot bath. Toss in about a cup of Epsom salt (also known as magnesium sulfate). Slide down in the tub and soak for 15 to 20 minutes. Yes, that's recovery. Magnesium sulfate has been shown to help muscles relax and reduce inflammation—just what they need after a tough workout.

HOW IT HELPS: Epsom salt is a strong vasodilator, which means it increases blood-flow to the muscles as well as to the surface of the skin. Epsom salt baths will also help rid your body of toxins and impurities by increasing perspiration.

What's more, magnesium is absorbed through the skin, which increases levels of magnesium in the blood. Magnesium helps build bones, manufacture proteins, release energy from muscles, and regulate body temperature, among other benefits. We bet you'll never look at a hot bath the same way again—all those benefits from relaxing in a hot tub are hard to beat.

HOW MUCH/HOW OFTEN: Ideally, soak 2 or 3 times per week.

HOW TO USE IT: Fill your tub with the hottest water you can stand (to promote sweating) and add 1 to 1½ cups of Epsom salt. You want to saturate the water in the tub, so play with the amount of salt until you get enough so that just a few grains are left in the bottom of your bathwater—this is just past the point of saturation. A good rule of thumb is that a 4-pound container of salt (which looks like a half-gallon carton of milk) will give you 3 or 4 baths. If you like, add 2 or 3 drops of essential oil (lavender, eucalyptus, peppermint, or chamomile). Soak for 15 to 30 minutes. Afterward, take a cool shower to wash off the sweat-out toxins and remove excess salt from your skin.

DR. BROOKE SAYS: I often tell my patients to turn down the lights, light a candle, and sip a champagne glass of sparkling water—it's a nice indulgence. Or drink a hot cup of chamomile tea as you soak—it's relaxing and really gets you sweating.

R&R Tool #5: Ice Massage

Formally known as cryotherapy, ice massage is another readily accessible and inexpensive recovery technique.

HOW IT HELPS: Ice massage is extremely effective for reducing inflammation. The cold makes the blood vessels in the tissue contract, which reduces circulation. When you remove the source of the cold, the blood vessels overcompensate and dilate, and blood rushes into the muscle, bringing with it the necessary nutrients to allow muscle healing.

HOW MUCH/HOW OFTEN: Ice massage therapy is most effective if it is applied soon after a workout. Incorporate this practice after very strenuous training sessions.

HOW TO USE IT: Fill paper cups with water and freeze. When you're ready for your ice massage, simply peel down the sides of a cup to expose more ice while performing the massage.

Gently massage the muscles in a circular motion for 5 to 10 minutes. *Note:* To avoid damaging the skin, do not let the ice sit on a particular area of skin for too long. If your skin is sensitive, use a gel or salve on the targeted area to provide a protective barrier for the skin.

DR. BROOKE SAYS: Don't use petroleum jelly to protect your skin from ice. I recommend Alba Multi-Purpose Un-Petroleum Jelly, Jason Tea Tree Oil Therapeutic Mineral Gel, or Traumeel from Heel. You'll find them at most natural foods stores and at www.bodybyhardware.com.

R&R Tool #6: Hot-and-Cold Contrasts

Alternating between hot and cold baths or showers can improve recovery dramatically, especially after an intense training session.

HOW IT HELPS: Hot baths will increase the peripheral bloodflow toward the skin and muscles, while cold plunges will force the body to redirect that bloodflow back toward the internal organs. This technique of external to internal bloodflow will facilitate the removal of metabolic waste products from the tissues.

HOW MUCH/HOW OFTEN: Ideally, you'd incorporate this into your daily shower, but at the very least, you should include contrasts after an intense training session.

HOW TO USE IT: First, you need to know what we mean by "hot" and "cold." Hot temperature ranges from 95° to 104°F, while cold temperature ranges from 50° to 60°F. Since you probably won't carry a thermometer into the bath or shower, simply use your best judgment—and take care not to scald your skin!

- **In the shower:** Get under a hot, steamy spray for 1 to 2 minutes. Then gather your courage and turn the water to cold. Stand under the cold water for 30 to 60 seconds. Alternate between the hot/cold spray 3 or 4 times.

- **In the bath:** Immerse your body in cold water for 30 to 60 seconds. Then get out of the bath and towel dry for 60 seconds. Repeat 3 or 4 times.

DR. BROOKE SAYS: Work up to a cold plunge. First immerse your hands and feet. With each shower, work your way up to splashing more of your body with cold water. After perhaps five or six times, you are ready to go full blast. And include your head and face—the cold water will make your skin glow!

R&R Tool #7: Sauna Therapy

Many people think of sauna therapy as a tool for athletes who train intensely, but the fact is, it's also an excellent tool for nonathletes: Taking a sauna can help your muscles recover, too. If your health club has a sauna, we highly recommend making use of it.

HOW IT HELPS: Some of the benefits of regular sauna use include the following: increased bloodflow to the peripheral tissues, removal of toxins, and relaxation of the muscular and nervous systems.

HOW MUCH/HOW OFTEN: Visit a sauna as often as your schedule allows, the morning after your cheat meal (especially if it includes alcohol), and whenever you need some downtime. Don't exceed more than five sessions per week.

HOW TO USE IT: If you use the sauna, follow these important guidelines.

- The best time to take a sauna is 1 to 2 hours after you train, rather than immediately following your workout. But if your schedule doesn't allow you to return to the gym later in the day, it's fine to step into the sauna immediately after your workout.

- Before you enter the sauna, shower with soap and dry your skin. This creates the optimal environment for sweat release and thermal regulation.

- As for the actual usage, two or three 10-minute exposures to the sauna followed by a brief (i.e., 30- to 60-second) cooldown shower (water temperature should be about 70°F) in between each exposure provides optimal recovery benefits.

DR. BROOKE SAYS: For the first "round," stay in the sauna until you break a really good sweat. For some people, that can take 10 minutes or more. After that, alternate between hot/cold in 10-minute intervals.

R&R Tool #8: Massage Therapy

Though costly, massage therapy provides numerous benefits and feels heavenly. If you can afford it, go for it! If not, no worries—foam rolling is an inexpensive yet effective alternative.

HOW IT HELPS: Massage therapy will:

- Help relax the nervous system and reduce your stress levels

- Help relax muscle spasms and release muscular tension

- Aid the lymphatic system in its function of releasing excess fluids from tissue and improving immune system function

- Improve oxygen and nutrient supply to the muscles, tendons, and ligaments and aid in the removal of metabolic waste because of its positive effect on the circulatory system

HOW MUCH/HOW OFTEN: Include massages as often as your finances and schedule allow. Every other week is ideal.

DR. BROOKE SAYS: States require that practitioners be certified as LMPs (licensed massage practitioners), and many have advanced certificates or specialties. But it's fine to drop in at your local nail salon and get a quick, cheap massage for your upper shoulders as often as you can. It's less technically effective than a rubdown given by an LMP but still easy, inexpensive, and relaxing.

R&R Tool #9: Recovery Pool Work

Another excellent recovery technique is active recovery work in a pool.

HOW IT HELPS: Water has a therapeutic effect on the body and mind. It provides both buoyancy, which allows for an unloading of body weight, and resistance, which allows for training with minimal impact on the body.

HOW MUCH/HOW OFTEN: Ideally, you'll use the pool for 10 to 20 minutes the day after a heavy training session, with a very light to moderate intensity.

HOW TO USE IT: Stick to walking, jogging, treading water, basic swimming strokes, and stretching. These are the activities best suited for pool work.

DR. BROOKE SAYS: If you have lower-back problems, pool work is an excellent tool. Any swimming stroke will unload the spine because you are not vertical and compressing your spine/disks.

FOAM ROLLING IN 8 EASY MOVES

Think of a foam roller as the poor man's masseuse. After a hard workout, a few minutes with the roller can be a simple and soothing reward. Basically, you position muscles across the roller and use it—and your body weight—to massage them, reducing soreness and increasing flexibility.

Your gym may have foam rollers you can use. If not, they're available at sporting goods stores or online for as little as $20 (see Resources in the Appendix). Foam rollers come in 1- to 3-foot lengths. You can buy a shorter roller for traveling and a long one for your workout space if you train at home. Purchase the rollers made of "molded foam," if possible. These maintain their density without flattening out over time. We prefer the 1-foot by 6-inch model, which can be purchased at www.performbetter.com and www.bodybyhardware.com.

In our foam-rolling sequence, you'll hit 8 knot-prone areas, from calves to spine. You'll spend 30 seconds on each area—more if you find a sore, tender spot. If you don't feel any, that's great, but spend 30 seconds on that muscle anyway. As you roll, be mindful of head and spinal alignment.

Please don't skip foam rolling. The better your tissue quality and length, the less likely you are to get injured and the better your training will progress. The entire sequence takes less than 10 minutes. Joe's had clients tell him that once they start doing it, they may roll for 15 or 20 minutes because it feels so good!

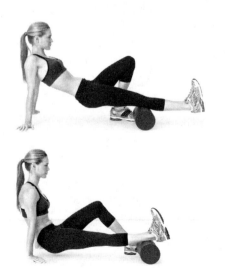

1. **Calves:** Sit with the roller under your right calf. Place the palms of your hands on the ground, fingers pointing toward your body. Keep your chest up and your spine in good alignment. Keep your left foot off the ground by stacking your feet on top of each other (heel of left foot on toe of right foot). Supporting your body weight on your hands, roll up and down along your calf. First, roll back and forth with your calf in a neutral position, then externally rotate your calf slightly to hit the outer muscles. Next, turn your calf in and roll the inner part. Repeat on your other calf.

2. **Hamstrings:** Sit with the roller under your right thigh. Place your palms on the ground, fingers pointing toward your body. Supporting your body weight with your hands, roll up and down from the bottom of your hip bone to the top of your knees. First roll back and forth with the leg in a neutral position, then externally rotate your leg slightly to hit the outer hamstring muscles. Next, turn your leg in and roll the inner part of your hamstring. Repeat on your other hamstring.

3. **Glutes:** Sit with one glute on the roller, crossing that leg and resting your foot on the opposite knee. Leaning slightly on that glute, roll from underneath the glute to the back of your hip bone. Roll back to the starting position. Roll back and forth for at least 30 seconds, rolling with your foot turned in and out to cover the entire muscle group. Repeat on the other glute. You can increase or reduce pressure by using one or both legs at a time.

4. **Iliotibial (IT) band:** The IT band is a thick band of connective tissue that runs along the outside of the thigh. It begins at the hip and extends to the outer side of the shinbone (tibia) just below the knee joint. The band works with several muscles in the thigh to stabilize the outside of the knee joint. It's a tender area for many people—especially runners—and a major source of knee problems.

   Lie on one side. Extend your bottom leg straight out. Cross your top leg over your bottom leg. Place the foam roller just above the joint of your bottom knee but on the lateral aspect of your thigh. Using your bottom elbow to move your body, slowly roll up and down your outer thigh from below your hip bone to just above your knee. Turn your leg in to roll the inner knee, and then outward to roll the outer part. Roll over and repeat on the other side.

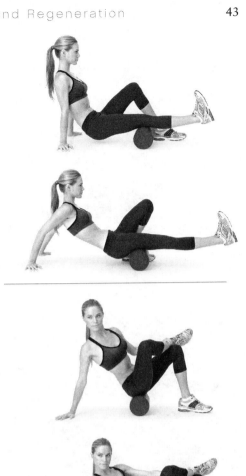

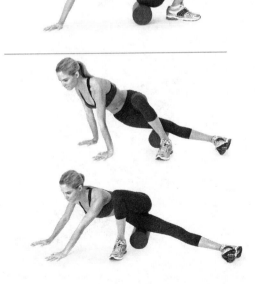

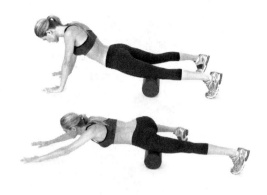

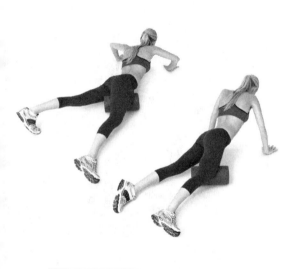

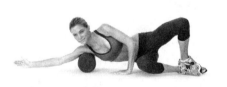

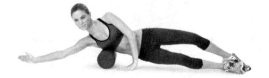

5. **Quads:** Lie facedown with the foam roller under your right thigh, just above the kneecap. Use your arms for balance. Keep your left foot off the ground by stacking your feet on top of each other (toe of left foot on heel of right foot). Supporting your body weight with your hands or forearms, roll up and down from the bottom of the hip to the top of your knee. Roll with your leg in a neutral position several times. Turn your leg in to roll the inner quad, and then outward to roll the outer quad. Repeat on your other quad.

6. **Adductor:** The muscles of the inner thigh run from the inner knee up into the groin. You may get some strange looks performing this one, but it's important.

   Lie facedown on the floor; come up and balance on your hands or forearms. Place the roller perpendicular to your body. Extend the leg opposite the roller straight out, thigh and knee down. Place your other leg—the one closest to the roller—over the roller so that it's under your inner thigh. Inching your body sideways, roll the inside of your leg all the way down until just inside your knee. Roll back toward the hip. Switch legs and repeat.

7. **Lats:** Like the IT band, many people find this area to be very tender, and foam rolling will iron out those knots. Lie on your side; extend your bottom arm away from your body. Place the roller horizontally, just below your pectoral (chest) muscles. Roll up just past your shoulder and armpit, then back.

   As you roll, experiment with tilting your torso slightly forward or back to zero in on tender spots. Tilt forward and you'll hit your pectoral muscles. Tilt back and you'll hit some of the back shoulder muscles, which tend to be sore as well.

8. **Thoracic spine (T spine):** If you sit in front of a computer all day, this one is going to feel really good. The T spine often becomes hunched from sitting in front of a computer and is a major cause of neck and shoulder pain.

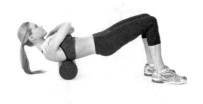

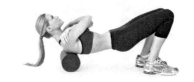

Lie on your back; cross your arms across your chest as if you're giving yourself a hug. (This moves your shoulder blades out of the way so the roller can get to the muscles around the spine.) Draw your feet in toward your butt with your knees off the floor, so they point at the ceiling. Place the roller under your midback.

Lift your hips off the floor and roll toward the top of the back—stop before you reach your neck—and back down to your midback. Continue to roll back and forth, from midback to just below your neck to midback.

STATIC STRETCHING SEQUENCE

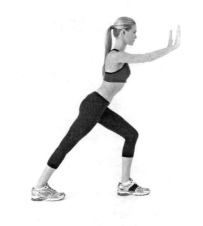

1. **Standing Calf Stretch (Gastroc):** Stand in front of a wall or some other vertical support. Place both hands on the support about chest level. Take a step back so that you are in a staggered stance and the heel of your trail leg is about 3 to 4 feet from the wall. The knee of your front leg should be bent, and the knee of your trail leg should be fully extended with your foot flat on the floor. While keeping your heel down, slowly lean forward to increase the stretch. Repeat on the other side.

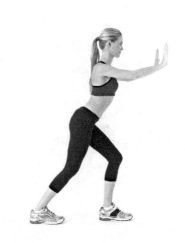

2. **Standing Calf Stretch (Soleus):** Stand in front of a wall or some other vertical support. Place both hands on the support about chest level. Take a step back so that you are in a staggered stance and the heel of your trail leg is about 2 to 3 feet from the wall. The knee of your front leg should be bent, and the knee of your trail leg should also be bent with your foot flat on the floor. While keeping your heel down, slowly lean forward to increase the stretch. Repeat on the other side.

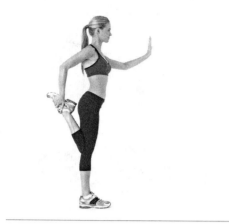

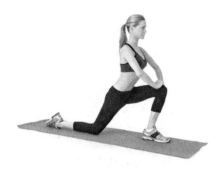

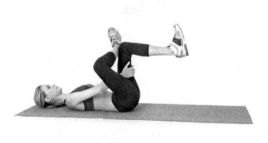

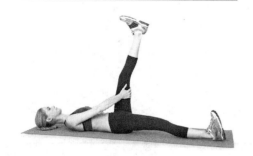

3. **Standing Quad Stretch:** Stand in front of a wall or some other vertical support. Place your left hand on the wall, and grab your right foot with your right hand and gently pull your heel toward your butt. Make sure you maintain a tall spine. To increase the stretch, you can slowly push your hips forward. Repeat on the other side.

4. **Kneeling Hip Flexor Stretch:** Assume a kneeling split-squat position so that the shin of your lead leg and the thigh of your trail leg are in a vertical position. The foot of your lead leg should be flat on the floor, and the knee of your trail leg should be on the floor with your toes in contact with the floor. (You may place a small towel or pad under your knee for comfort.) Slowly push your hips forward while keeping your torso in an upright position. Repeat on the other side.

5. **Lying Glute Stretch:** Lie on your back with your hips and knees bent. Cross your right leg so that your right ankle is resting against your left leg just above your knee. With your hands, reach between your legs and grab the back of your left leg just below the knee. Slowly pull your left leg toward your chest while simultaneously trying to keep the shin and knee of your right leg perpendicular to your left leg. Repeat on the other side.

6. **Lying Hamstring Stretch:** Lie on your back and raise your right leg as high as you can while keeping it straight. Take both hands and grab behind your right thigh and gently pull it further toward your torso. Make sure you keep your butt on the ground; your opposite leg should remain straight—try not to let it rotate outward. (You can also place a towel around your foot and pull gently toward your torso.) Repeat on the other side.

7. **Bent-Over Lat Stretch:** Stand in front of an incline bench (or any sturdy upright structure, such as a door frame) and grab the top of the bench with both hands. Your arms should be outstretched; your torso should be either parallel or slightly above parallel to the floor, with your knees slightly bent and your butt back. Slowly shift your hips slightly to the left side while keeping a firm grip on the bench. Next, shift your hips to the right side.

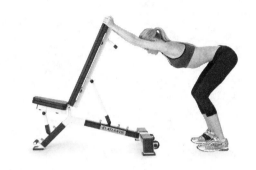

8. **Half-Kneeling Pec Stretch:** Assume a half-kneeling stance alongside an incline bench (or any sturdy upright structure, such as a door frame). Bend your elbow to a 90° angle and place your elbow and forearm against the bench. Make sure your upper arm is parallel or slightly below parallel to the floor. Begin by slowly rotating your torso away from the bench. Repeat on the other side.

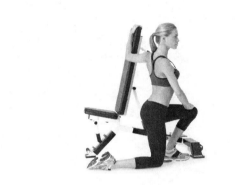

9. **Standing Triceps Stretch:** While standing, raise your right arm above your head and maximally bend your elbow so that your right hand is touching your upper back between your shoulder blades. Now, take your left hand and reach up and over your head and grab behind the elbow of your right arm; gently pull the right arm backward. Repeat on the other side.

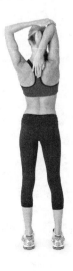

CHAPTER 5

How Your Hormonal Landscape Affects Your Weight

EVERY DAY, EVERY MEAL, EVERY hour—every minute, actually—you have an opportunity to encourage your body to burn fat or to store it.

Will you eat breakfast or skip it? Select a salad for lunch or a slice of pizza? Turn in before midnight or pull an all-nighter? Obsess over a troubled relationship or soothe yourself with a warm bath or a walk? These choices can profoundly affect your body's internal chemistry, which can, in turn, influence your physique.

Every day, every meal, every hour—every minute, actually—you have an opportunity to encourage your body to burn fat or to store it.

If you expect to count calories, carbs, or fat grams, this program will come as a welcome surprise. On the Ultimate You program, you manage your body's hormonal responses to foods, eating (or not eating), sleep, stress, and exercise. To help your body utilize food more efficiently, avoid cravings, and increase your body's ability to burn fat, you need a working knowledge of your internal chemistry and your hormones.

Hormones are your body's chemical messengers. They travel in your bloodstream to tissues or organs. They affect many different processes, including sexual function, reproduction, mood, internal balance of body systems (homeostasis), and metabolism—how the body gets energy from food.

This chapter discusses the hormones that affect metabolism. Until recently, the role of hormones in fat loss has been largely ignored in favor of the "calories in, calories out" model.

FROM "EAT LESS, MOVE MORE" TO "EAT BETTER, MOVE SMARTER"

In the traditional view of weight loss—let's call it the eat-less-move-more (ELMM) model—the body is like a bank account. "Spend" (burn) more calories than you "save" (consume) and you lose weight.

In reality, the body is more like a chemistry lab, and weight loss is more complex than the ELMM model implies. Yes, if you reduce calories, you'll often lose some weight. But "losing weight" alone doesn't achieve an Ultimate You physique. To get that, you have to lose fat, not just weight, and "eat less, move more" doesn't work for fat loss, which requires a unique hormonal "landscape."

On the Ultimate You program, you eat better and move smarter.

On the Ultimate You program, you eat better and move smarter. "Eat better" means you know what to eat and when, and you pay less attention to calories than to the quality of what you put in your mouth (fresh, natural, whole foods rather than processed junk and too many simple carbs). As you'll learn, all calories are not created equal, and the calories you choose can significantly impact how much fat your body burns or stores.

Here's an example: A large chocolate-chip cookie contains around 190 calories. So does ¼ cup of dry-roasted cashews. No difference, calorie-wise. But the nutrients they contain are worlds apart. The cashews provide healthy, monounsaturated fats; minerals such as copper, magnesium, and phosphorus; and fiber. The cookie provides sugar and not much else.

More important, each of these foods sends a different hormonal "message." The cashews send a message of satisfaction and satiety, while the insulin spike from the cookie sends the message to store fat. The point: To lose fat, focus less on calories and more on foods' effect on your hormones.

HORMONES: THE METABOLIC MOTOR

The transformation of "weight loss" into fat loss begins at the cellular level. Each cell in your body—itself a tiny chemistry lab—determines your *metabolism*, the reactions

how do I know when it's my hormones?

When your hormones are unbalanced, your body can feel dreadful. You may also gain weight or have a hard time losing it.

There are many causes of hormonal imbalances, from a poor diet to toxins in the environment. However, having your hormones tested can be less helpful than you'd think. While overt hormone disorders show up on routine lab tests, more subtle "subclinical" disruptions, which can definitely affect physical and emotional well-being, might not.

More alternative methods, such as salivary or urine tests, can help better discern slight disruptions. But even they don't always indicate actual hormone activity in your body; thus, symptoms shouldn't be ignored. On this program, you will learn to correct many imbalances yourself by using your symptoms as a guide. Should you need more assistance, you'll find resources on how to find a practitioner that can help.

in cells that convert fuel from food into the energy the body needs to function—move, think, digest food, repair itself.

Your metabolism—and these ongoing processes—is governed by the endocrine system. The glands of this system, which include the thyroid, ovaries, pituitary, pancreas, and adrenals, release hormones directly into the bloodstream, where they are transported to cells in other parts of the body.

Your metabolism's mission is *balance*: the oscillation of repair and regeneration, as your body constantly breaks down old tissues and replaces them with new, healthier tissue. The constant ebb and flow as your body builds itself up and breaks itself down is known as *anabolism* and *catabolism*. When one hormone or hormonal pathway is out of balance, it is just a matter of time before another becomes imbalanced—and the resulting imbalances can impact the body's ability to burn fat.

In recent years, the role of hormones on fat loss has gained attention. Some diets stress managing the effects of insulin; others emphasize the control of cortisol. However, it's problematic to view any one hormone in isolation. To have a healthy metabolism, all hormones must be in perfect balance.

Often, in the discussion of weight, hormones are described as "good" or "bad." Hormones are neither—they simply encourage the body to burn or store fat, depending on the situation. For example, insulin's storage effects are ideal post-workout but not so good after a big dinner. And cortisol's ability to raise blood sugar is great during a tough workout but not great when it has to boost blood sugar because you skipped breakfast. The bottom line: There's a time and place for each hormone.

Our diet and lifestyle recommendations will help raise or lower hormones at the appropriate times. So, for example, cortisol will rise during the intense workouts we recommend; this is a signal to the body to release glucagon, growth hormone, and testosterone. These hormones trigger fat burning. After the workout, we're going to use a Recovery Shake that will help take advantage of insulin sensitivity post-workout to enhance recovery and shut off cortisol release. All of this will turn you into a lean, fat-burning machine. You don't need to memorize any of this—there won't be a test! Just know that we've designed every aspect of this program to balance your hormones and optimize results.

YOUR "I'M FULL" HORMONES: CCK AND LEPTIN

There are four major hormones that regulate appetite: ghrelin, neuropeptide Y, CCK (cholecystokinin), and leptin. Ghrelin and neuropeptide Y tell you that you are hungry; CCK and leptin tell you that you're full. All of these hormones can be manipulated through diet and lifestyle.

Secreted by intestinal cells (and perhaps the brain as well), CCK regulates short-term hunger. When you eat fiber and fat, CCK signals the release of digestive enzymes and bile (needed for fat absorption) and slows the emptying of your stomach. The result: Fat and fiber help you feel full.

Leptin deals more with long-term hunger, such as between meals and overnight. Secreted from your fat cells, leptin works like a gas gauge on your car: It tells your brain how full your tank is. When things are working properly, the message is "There's sufficient fat around, so you don't need to eat much, and it's fine to let go of some stores."

If your body is resistant to the effects of leptin, the "you're full" message is not heeded, and you experience more hunger more often.

The power to change your body is in your hands!

Here's the good news: Appropriate intake of fiber and good fat helps to regulate CCK; leptin can be controlled by meal-timing, lowering body fat, and sleep. That means that the power to change your body is in your hands!

INSULIN AND GLUCAGON: MAKING AND BREAKING FAT

The feather-shaped pancreas, near the liver, secretes these two important metabolic hormones. As an anabolic hormone, insulin builds up both sugar stores and fat stores by moving fuel out of the bloodstream. Glucagon, a catabolic hormone, breaks both of those stores down.

Take that information in: Insulin builds up fat stores, and glucagon breaks them down. On this program, you'll learn to minimize insulin to help you burn fat, maximize glucagon's ability to burn it, and take advantage of insulin's storage and recovery actions, which will be especially important post-workout.

Acting primarily on liver, muscle, and fat cells, insulin lowers blood sugar by increasing the body's stores of sugar and fat. Now, your body needs *some* stores of sugar and fat. Extra sugar in your muscles and liver ensures that you do not have to eat constantly to keep your blood sugar and energy up. Fat stores are necessary as well, although not in the quantity many people have.

Insulin sends a clear message to fat cells: Increase fat stores and stop burning fat. That's why many weight-loss experts recommend low-carb eating—it lowers insulin levels. But attempting to keep insulin low all of the time is a misguided approach to fat loss. The one time when high insulin levels pay off is after your workouts; in Phase 2, you'll learn how to use insulin to build up your reserves, enhance recovery, and mitigate the stress effect of a tough workout.

When fat, muscle, and liver cells are receptive to the actions of insulin, you are "sensitive" to insulin's message. When you are insulin *resistant*, your cells ignore insulin's message, so your pancreas secretes more and more of the hormone in an effort to be heard. Left unchecked, insulin resistance will increase fat stores. Worse, it often leads to type 2 diabetes. The good news: If you're insulin resistant, this program may well help you reverse the condition.

Let's move on to glucagon. While insulin lowers blood sugar, this hormone raises it. Glucagon breaks down glycogen (stored sugar) in response to either a decline in blood sugar (and low insulin) or the presence of adrenaline, lactic acid, or amino acids from dietary protein. This is one reason you'll eat a lot of lean protein on this plan: It opposes insulin's "store fat" message and encourages your body to burn it.

could you be insulin resistant?

You may be—at least to some degree—if you answer yes to any of the questions below.

- Do you get sleepy after meals?
- Do you have a ravenous appetite most of the time?
- Do you live to eat rather than eat to live?
- Do protein foods like meat and fish give you energy?
- Do vegetarian meals tend to not satisfy you?
- Do you crave something sweet immediately after eating a meal of protein and veggies?

- Do you get hungry between meals?
- Do you feel poorly when you try to do a fast?
- Do you tend to store fat around your midsection or along your bra line?
- Have you been diagnosed with type 2 diabetes, metabolic syndrome, or polycystic ovarian syndrome (PCOS)?
- Have you been diagnosed with any of the following: elevated fasting blood glucose/sugar, elevated cholesterol or triglycerides, high blood sugar, or a waist-to-hip ratio of greater than 0.7?

Another thing that stimulates glucagon production: intense exercise. Typically, weight-loss experts recommend moderate-intensity workouts. The Ultimate You workouts are not too long and are intense enough to trigger an almost magic scenario where glucagon, cortisol, growth hormone, and lactic acid join forces to burn fat.

To burn fat, you must manage your body's ratio of insulin secretion to glucagon secretion. To do that, you'll learn how to control what you eat and when you eat it. For example, a meal higher in carbohydrates will cause the pancreas to secrete more insulin, while a higher-protein meal will induce a more balanced ratio of insulin to glucagon.

Further, when your blood sugar dips between meals, glucagon allows your body to tap into stored fat. That's why you won't nibble every 2 hours, as other weight-loss plans recommend. When you eat that often, your body releases insulin constantly, all through the day—not good, if you're trying to burn fat.

But no worries—you won't go too long without food. (That puts a damper on your body's ability to burn fat as well.) On your way to becoming your Ultimate You, you'll know exactly when you'll eat your next meal or snack.

CORTISOL: MALIGNED AND MISUNDERSTOOD

Poor cortisol: It means well but just doesn't know when to quit. Produced by the adrenal glands, this catabolic (breakdown) hormone is released in response to any stress, including cold, fasting, infection, pain, intense exercise, and lack of sleep.

We couldn't survive without cortisol—and yet this stress hormone is unfairly blamed for thickened waistlines and bulging bellies. In fact, some of its actions favor leanness (more on that later). The problem: Constant, unremitting stress can keep this survival mechanism churning in high gear, subverting cortisol's good intentions. What's more, cortisol doesn't act alone. It's aided and abetted by the fat-storing hormone insulin.

Here's the deal. As a "stress hormone," cortisol helps you tap into your energy reserves—stored sugar, fat, and protein (in the form of muscle tissue) during a crisis, whether perceived or real.

Cortisol is released in a cyclic manner; levels should be highest in the early morning, decline gradually through the day, and be lowest by bedtime. Constant stress, however, disrupts this cycle. The result: Cortisol is released continuously, along with another important stress hormone, adrenaline.

These hormones raise your blood sugar so you have the fuel you need to react to a life-threatening event—a survival mechanism that dates back to our caveman ancestors. The vast majority of their stressors were life threatening and necessitated intense physical activity. It requires a lot of fuel to either fight off or outrun a wild animal!

Most 21st-century stresses don't require you to fight or flee, which means they don't require fuel. Alas, they still raise your blood levels of sugar and fat. Chronic stress *not* followed by physical activity increases the body's fat stores, particularly in the belly. What's more, the release

belly fat: more than maddening

A big belly threatens more than your self-esteem: It threatens your health.

Belly fat produces substances called cytokines that can cause chronic inflammation, which in turn promotes heart disease and type 2 diabetes. Its close proximity to your vital organs, including your liver, kidneys, heart, and lungs, makes that inflammation pretty scary. What's more, belly-fat cells actually make more cortisol—perpetuating the pooch.

People who don't manage cortisol well tend to store more belly fat. These "apple-shaped" folks have a higher risk of heart disease and diabetes.

Lose the belly and you won't just look better—you'll significantly lower your risk of cardiovascular disease and diabetes. Belly fat is often the last area of fat to go, so don't give up. Stay on plan, be consistent—and don't stress about it.

of cortisol is followed by a release of insulin. This constant release of cortisol and insulin places your body in constant fat-storing mode.

Fortunately, lifestyle changes—sound nutrition, regular exercise, stress management—can help you gain control of your cortisol levels and your weight.

ESTROGEN: THE HORMONE OF FEMININITY—AND FAT

Produced in the ovaries, this female sex hormone is the essence of femininity, the bestower of smooth skin and curvy hips. As an anabolic hormone that builds up bone, the uterine lining, and body fat, estrogen also regulates the menstrual cycle and protects the heart and bones.

However, in excess, this otherwise beneficial hormone can endanger a woman's health and wreak havoc on her physique. In a relatively high estrogen state, known as *estrogen dominance*, women can really pack on the pounds, particularly in the hips, thighs, and butt. Further, because estrogen dominance can worsen insulin resistance, estrogen-dominant women tend to store fat around their waists. (To see if you might be estrogen dominant, take the quiz on the opposite page.)

Perimenopause and menopause can cause estrogen dominance, too. This may sound odd, given that both conditions are characterized by low levels of estrogen. But while estrogen may be overtly low, it can still dominate progesterone and testosterone.

The source of this excess estrogen isn't the ovaries—it's medications such as birth control pills and our environment. Both compounds that occur naturally and man-made chemicals in our air, water, and food—everything from plastic water bottles and shampoo to pesticides on fruits and veggies—contain molecules called *endocrine disruptors*, which research shows affect our health. Today, girls get their first periods at younger and younger ages. Estrogen-related cancers of the breast and uterus, as well as estrogen-related conditions such as fibroids and endometriosis, are on the rise. Estrogen dominance can also cause severe PMS, PCOS (polycystic ovarian syndrome), acne, and difficult perimenopause.

Endocrine disruptors block the effects of hormones that balance estrogen's effects, which causes estrogen to dominate a woman's hormonal landscape. For example, endocrine disruptors can lower the effects of progesterone and testosterone by blocking

could you be estrogen dominant?

If you answer yes to any of the questions below, it's likely that estrogen plays a role in your weight issues.

- Are you overweight?
- Do you carry body fat in your hips and thighs?
- Have you ever been pregnant?
- Do you have a hypothyroid condition?
- Do you have fibroids, endometriosis, or PCOS?
- Have you taken or do you currently take birth control pills?
- Have you taken or do you currently take synthetic hormone replacement (HRT)?
- Do you eat a lot of phytoestrogenic foods, such as soy?
- Are you menopausal or perimenopausal?

SOY FOODS AND "FEMALE HERBS": EASY DOES IT

Phytoestrogens are naturally occurring plant substances that have hormone-like activity. Examples of phytoestrogens are genistein and daidzein, found in soy and soy products. Some herbs have estrogenic activity as well.

Chemically, phytoestrogens resemble estrogen and usually have weak estrogenic activity. However, in a body already overloaded with estrogen, adding more can contribute to the problem.

Soy foods include soybeans, soy milk, tofu, tempeh, textured vegetable protein, roasted soybeans, soy protein powders, miso, and edamame. The lignans in flaxseed and herbs such as red clover, black cohosh, Vitex (chasteberry), and dong quai also have estrogenic activity.

Consuming a soy-heavy diet or taking phytoestrogenic herbs for a long period of time can significantly impact estrogen dominance. Some phytoestrogens have also been shown to hinder thyroid function.

Because of its strong hormonal action and its tendency to cause digestive upset, limit your intake of soy. If you have a thyroid condition, avoid it completely. Use the herbs listed above with supervision of a healthcare provider to ensure you aren't tipping the scales in favor of estrogen dominance.

their production by the adrenal glands. Endocrine disruptors also can act as strong estrogens themselves.

As you might guess, endocrine disruptors affect women more than men. (While men can be estrogen dominant, their higher levels of testosterone and greater muscle mass have a protective effect.)

Estrogen dominance is frustrating but fixable. You'll learn about foods and supplements that can help reduce estrogen dominance in Phase 3.

PROGESTERONE: THE "OTHER FEMALE HORMONE"

Estrogen fills out a woman's hips and thighs; progesterone nips her waist. A woman's classic hourglass shape is the happy result of balanced levels of estrogen and progesterone.

Produced in the ovaries, the adrenal glands, and in the placenta when a woman gets pregnant, progesterone helps prepare a woman's body for conception and pregnancy and regulates the monthly menstrual cycle. It also plays a role in mood, appetite,

everyday estrogens

Endocrine disruptors—substances in pesticides, herbicides, some plastics, and even our air and water—can add to the body's estrogen burden. So can xenoestrogens—manmade compounds that have unintended estrogen effects. The scary part: You're exposed to them every day.

You can't avoid all of these substances. But if you know where they lurk, you can limit your exposure to at least some of them. Here's a list of significant sources of these health-threatening chemicals.

Common Endocrine Disruptors

- Cosmetics (phthalates and parabens), air fresheners, flooring (phthalates)

- Plastic bottles and containers, linings of some metal cans (bisphenol A)

- Flame retardants in bedding (polybrominated diphenyl ethers)

- Styrofoam (dioxins)

Common Xenoestrogens

- Commercially raised meat
- Canned foods
- Plastics, plastic food wraps
- Styrofoam cups
- Industrial wastes
- Car exhaust and indoor toxins
- Pesticides and herbicides
- Paints, lacquers, and solvents
- Personal-care products
- Cosmetics
- Birth control pills and spermicide
- Hormone replacement therapy drugs
- Detergents
- All artificial scents (air fresheners, perfumes, etc.)
- Carpet fibers
- Teflon coating on nonstick cookware

sleep quality, memory, and sexual desire and negates some of the unfavorable effects of estrogen on the breasts and uterus.

Progesterone also has a significant impact on a woman's ability to lose body fat. Progesterone promotes leanness by countering the fat-storing effect of cortisol at the belly and estrogen at the hips.

Alas, chronic stress reduces progesterone levels. Progesterone is a parent hormone, which means it has its own actions *and* can be converted into other hormones, including cortisol. When you are constantly in fight-or-flight mode, your adrenal glands will need to produce additional cortisol.

The problem: When you are under constant stress, the demands for cortisol are great enough that your adrenals convert progesterone into more cortisol. In a process known as the progesterone steal, your body will steal however much progesterone it needs to make cortisol. (If, during a time of stress, your menstrual flow was lighter than usual or you skipped your period entirely, you've experienced the progesterone steal.) So when cortisol dominates your hormonal landscape, it's easy to pack on progesterone-deficient padding.

TESTOSTERONE: NOT JUST FOR BOYS

As a woman, you don't make a lot of this male sex hormone, but the little you do make is critical to your health and well-being. As it does for men, testosterone helps women feel confident, think clearly, and feel lusty. It has widespread anabolic effects on muscle, organs, bone marrow (where it helps make red blood cells), and skin, where it stimulates growth and repair of tissues.

Testosterone also helps women stay lean by helping to block cortisol's fat-storing message to belly fat. A woman's testosterone levels decline both with age and with extra pounds. As testosterone dips, women have a harder and harder time losing body fat.

Many women are low in testosterone even by female standards, often due to improper diet and exercise habits (i.e., low protein intake, excessive cardio, and not lifting weights), lack of sleep, stress, or estrogen dominance. While testosterone/estrogen balance is largely responsible for female leanness overall, low testosterone specifically causes less-than-toned arms and that flab between the breasts and

growth hormone: testosterone's sidekick

Testosterone and growth hormone work together and are essential if you want to get lean.

Secreted from the anterior pituitary gland in your brain, growth hormone promotes the growth of bone, muscle, and most organs. Normally, this hormone spikes every 4 hours and rises overnight as a response to fasting during sleep. When it comes to metabolism, it frees fat from fat cells for the muscle and heart to use as fuel while it helps get glucose to the brain, with the aid of cortisol. Growth hormone also helps muscle cells utilize dietary protein.

The take-home message: In the pres-ence of high enough growth hormone, you will burn fat over sugar. Basically, the more growth hormone you have, the leaner you are.

Growth hormone replacement therapy, along with a very low-calorie diet, is one of the latest weight-loss fads—some plans claim you can lose up to 3 pounds a day. If that sounds too good to be true, you're right. Such plans can wreak havoc on other hormones, which creates poorer health in the long run. Intense exercise, sleep, adequate protein, and management of stress are much better ways to raise this important hormone.

armpits. If the back of your arms continues to jiggle after you wave good-bye, if you've got fat bubbling out the side of your bra, or if you have any of the following symptoms, you may be at least relatively low in testosterone:

- Apathy/depression
- Anxiety
- Decreased stamina and endurance with exercise
- Inability to make clear decisions
- Insomnia
- Irritability
- Low libido or difficulty having an orgasm
- Poor memory/low concentration
- Poor recovery from illness and injury
- Weight gain, especially around the chest and middle

While low testosterone is a problem for any woman with too much body fat, it becomes a huge problem with the onset of menopause. When your overall sex-hormone production declines as ovaries shut down, you are left with just your adrenals to make progesterone and testosterone. And after decades of stress, those adrenals are tired! No worries, though—it's possible for you to raise your testosterone level with exercise, enough dietary protein, and sleep. You'll get the specifics in Phase 3.

LAST BUT NOT LEAST: THE THYROID

This small, butterfly-shaped gland sits in the throat, just above the collarbone. In adults, the thyroid's main action is to regulate the body's metabolic rate. No doubt about it: To burn fat, you need a healthy thyroid.

There are three main hormones associated with the thyroid: TSH (thyroid-stimulating hormone), T4, and T3. Secreted from the pituitary gland in the brain, TSH tells the thyroid gland to release T4 (and a bit of T3). T4 travels through the bloodstream and is converted to T3 (primarily in the liver). Once T3 reaches tissues such as cells in the digestive tract, liver, or muscle, the metabolism revs up.

There are more than 20 documented ways this system can get unbalanced—a lot of room for trouble. Too much of these hormones (hyperthyroidism) and your metabolism will speed up too much. More commonly, there's too little of these hormones (hypothyroidism) and metabolism slows down. There are more than 30 signs and symptoms of a sluggish thyroid. The most common are:

- Fatigue, even after a good night's sleep, or a mid-afternoon slump
- Lower-than-normal body temperature (98.6°F)
- Cold hands and feet
- Depression and mood swings
- Thinning hair
- Loss of outer ends of eyebrow lines
- Water retention
- Puffy eyelids, especially in the morning
- Dry skin

think you have a thyroid problem?

There are many symptoms related to hypothyroidism, from infertility to digestive issues. But if you have vague, unresolved ailments, struggle with weight loss, or experience any of the classic hypothyroid symptoms (see page 61), get your thyroid tested.

Most physicians will routinely test only your TSH levels. Ask for the additional tests below—they will help show the real picture.

- TSH
- Free T4 and total T4
- Free T3 and total T3
- Thyroid-binding globulin
- Reverse T3
- T3 uptake
- Anti-TPO and anti-thyroglobulin antibodies

As anyone diagnosed with hypothyroidism knows, this condition causes frustrating weight gain or makes it nearly impossible to lose weight.

Hypothyroidism is frequently underdiagnosed and often mismanaged. Diagnosis is typically done via blood tests. However, a TSH test is often the only screen performed, which often misses low levels of T3 and T4.

What's more, the American College of Endocrinology recently recommended an upper limit of 3.0 for TSH (rather than the typical 4.5 or 5.5). Yet not all physicians heed its recommendation.

What this means is that women who experience low-thyroid symptoms ask their doctors to test their thyroid and are found to have "normal" levels of TSH. They continue to struggle to lose weight, feel extreme fatigue, and experience many of the symptoms associated with low thyroid function. They're in the "undiagnosed club," often referred to as subclinical hypothyroidism.

Other women are diagnosed with hypothyroidism and treated with medications that act on T4 only, such as Synthroid or Levoxyl, yet continue to experience symptoms. These women may be members of the "mismanaged club."

Regardless of which club you belong to, you'll take steps to improve your thyroid function in Phase 4. And if you think you have a thyroid issue, get thoroughly tested and treated as soon as possible.

your hormone cheat sheet

HORMONE	ANABOLIC ACTIONS (BUILDING YOU UP)	CATABOLIC ACTIONS (BREAKING YOU DOWN)	LIFESTYLE TRIGGERS
Cortisol	Stores fat particularly at belly (high insulin often accompanies high cortisol)	Uses proteins and stored sugar for energy Uses stored fats for energy	Stress (especially chronic), skipping meals, exercise, low-calorie dieting, lack of sleep, alcohol
Epinephrine (a.k.a. adrenaline)	—	Uses stored sugar for energy	Acute stress, skipping meals, stimulants (including caffeine), low-calorie dieting, refined sugar, overdoing cardiovascular exercise
Insulin	Builds up sugar stores from dietary carbs and proteins Builds up fat stores from dietary carbs and fats Builds up proteins from dietary amino acids	—	Eating carbohydrates; cortisol or adrenaline release will cause subsequent insulin release; glucagon is also secreted with insulin when we eat protein
Glucagon	Triggers building up of new sugar stores in liver	Breaks down stored sugar	Low blood sugar (i.e., between meals), intense exercise
Estrogen	Builds up subcutaneous fat stores Builds up uterine lining	—	Xenoestrogens, phytoestrogens, and endocrine disruptors from medication, pesticides, etc., in our environment and diet; body fat converts testosterone to estrogen
Testosterone	Utilizes fat and sugar for energy Builds up proteins	—	REM sleep, adequate protein intake, intense exercise and weight training, adequate growth hormone
Growth hormone (HGH)	Utilizes fat stores for energy Builds up proteins	—	REM sleep, adequate protein intake, not eating too often, intense exercise and weight training
Thyroid hormones (T4 and T3)	Utilizes fat and sugar for energy Builds up proteins	—	Cold temperatures, healthy (not excessive) stress levels, normal estrogen levels, adequate calorie intake

CHAPTER 6

Fueling the Ultimate You

THANKS TO MAGAZINES, TV, THE Internet, and well-meaning friends and family, you are likely awash in a sea of diet information: low fat, low carb, low calorie, high protein, raw foods, and on and on it goes. The Ultimate You nutrition plan is your lifeline: a whole-foods, nutritious, plant-based, protein-rich, and satisfying diet that is as easy to follow as it is effective.

When it comes to fat loss, smart exercise is important—and the right nutrition plan is crucial. Your fat loss will depend largely on your diet, especially when you first begin. Remember: At every meal you have a choice to encourage your body to either store fat or burn it. The hormonal effect of your food choices sends that message to your body. In Chapter 5, you were introduced to the key hormones involved in fat burning and fat storage—now you'll learn how to send fat-burning messages to your body with the Ultimate You nutrition plan. And best of all? You won't be walking around hungry.

BEYOND THE GOOD-CARB/BAD-CARB PARADIGM

Popular low-carb diets have bred two notions: The first is that carbohydrates are either "good" (whole grains) or "bad" (rice, potatoes, pasta). The second is that all proteins and fats are created equal.

Those notions are too simplistic. You don't eat "protein" or "fat" or "carbohydrate." (Collectively, they're called *macronutrients*.) You eat food, which is extremely chemically complex, and your body secretes hormones in response to the amount of protein, fat, and carbohydrate the food contains. So on this plan, you pay attention to how a food's macronutrient content can affect your hormonal landscape. What you'll learn may surprise you.

For example, beans and legumes are commonly categorized as proteins, and they do contain a fair amount. But legumes contain more carbs than protein. One cup of black beans contains 15 grams of protein and 41 grams of carbohydrate and thus causes a significant insulin response. That's why this plan classifies beans and legumes as a high-fiber starch, rather than a protein. As nongrain plant foods loaded with antioxidants and fiber, beans and legumes make our Optimal high-fiber starch list.

Here's another example: Almonds, and nuts in general, are often considered high-

rev up your fiber intake

It can be tough to get the Ultimate You plan's recommended 35 to 50 grams of fiber a day. A supplement can bolster your daily intake so that you can take full advantage of fiber's satiating power.

Opt for a vegetable- and fruit-based fiber that contains acacia, guar gum, and fruit pectin, rather than a grain-based supplement.

If possible, choose a product that also contains probiotics and digestive enzymes—thus, a product that supports digestion as it promotes fat loss. Ultimate Fiber (Hardware) and Primal Fiber 1, 2, or 3 (Poliquin Performance) all fit the bill, but there may be others at your health-food store.

To avoid digestive upset and bloating, follow the recommendations that follow.

Increase your supplement by 1 to 2 teaspoons per week until you hit at least 35 grams of fiber per day from a combination of diet and supplements.

- **Week 1:** Follow the nutrition plan and increase your vegetable intake.

- **Week 2:** Add 1 to 2 teaspoons of powdered fiber in water at bedtime.

- **Week 3 and beyond:** Add another 1 to 2 teaspoons 30 minutes before meals or as a snack until you reach 35 to 50 grams per day.

Eventually, a typical day might look like this: 1 teaspoon 30 minutes before a meal and/or 1 teaspoon as a snack, as well as 1 to 2 teaspoons at bedtime.

protein foods. But ¼ cup of almonds contains 7.6 grams of protein and 18 grams of fat. So this plan classifies nuts not as proteins but fats.

When you eat the Ultimate You way, you don't stress about "good carbs" or "bad carbs." You classify carbs by how much fiber they contain—and you'll pay attention to grain-based versus plant-based fibers. A high-plant diet satisfies hunger and offers loads of fiber, a crucial nutrient for weight loss and appetite control.

TO SLIM DOWN, FIBER UP

Fiber-rich foods are the unsung champs of weight loss. Research backs this up: A University of Minnesota study found that people who ate the most vegetables, fruits, and other fiber-rich foods lost 2 to 3 pounds more per month than those on lower-fiber diets. Another study found that women who ate 13 grams of fiber or less per day were 5 times as likely to be overweight as those who ate more.

Fiber slows down eating because it requires more chewing. And it boosts satiety. When you eat fiber-rich foods, your body releases CCK (a hunger hormone), which slows the emptying of your stomach so you feel fuller longer. A slower rise in blood sugar from fiber also keeps insulin from spiking, meaning you store less fat.

Fiber comes in two types: soluble or insoluble. You need both kinds for optimal digestive health, correct metabolic hormone balance, appetite control, and fat loss.

Soluble fiber interacts with water like a sponge: It soaks it up. This makes your stomach empty more slowly. At the same time, fiber causes a slower rise in blood sugar, which prevents a spike in insulin. Now, because you're satisfied and your blood sugar is on an even keel, you're better able to manage hunger and cravings.

Found in the cell walls of plants such as vegetables, *insoluble fiber* doesn't dissolve in water. It functions like a scouring pad in your digestive tract, adding bulk to bowel movements. It also feeds friendly, healthy intestinal bacteria.

Most nutrition experts advise eating more whole grains as a way to increase the fiber in your diet. But this plan's carbohydrate list contains no highly processed grain products, and the Optimal list contains no grains at all. That's because grain-based fiber sources carry a big carb load and generate a significant insulin response—not what you want when you are trying to lose fat.

The key is to opt for carbohydrate sources with good ratios of fiber to starch or carbohydrate. On this program, you'll get plenty of the fiber you want—mostly from vegetables and some fruits—without the excessive carbohydrates you don't.

PROTEIN: ESSENTIAL FOR LIFE

Protein has long been the centerpiece of a healthy diet. Our hunter-gatherer ancestors ate a diet of animal protein and vegetables and were lean, strong, and not plagued in the same way as we are by modern diseases such as diabetes, cancer, and heart disease.

Protein is essential for life, an integral part of every cell. It is needed to build and maintain skin, muscle, bones, and organs. Proteins are also used to make hormones, transport nutrients, maintain water balance, and support immune function.

> Consider high-quality, lean animal proteins like "premium unleaded fuel" for your high-performance vehicle.

For your body to build or maintain tissue, your food choices must contain essential amino acids in sufficient amounts. Animal proteins—meat, fish, poultry, eggs, and whey protein (from dairy)—contain the essential amino acids in the proportions needed. They are most definitely foods your body needs for peak health and performance. Consider high-quality, lean animal proteins like "premium unleaded fuel" for your high-performance vehicle.

don't cheap out on protein

You get what you pay for: Conventionally raised meats are often loaded with inflammatory chemicals and exogenous hormones like estrogen, which can thwart weight loss. So spend a little extra on quality meat, poultry, and fish and your health and weight will benefit.

When you shop for protein, keep these tips in mind.

- Choose beef, poultry, and fish labeled "free range," "cage free," "grass fed," and "no hormones or antibiotics added."

- If you choose beef that is not grass fed, opt for the leanest cut possible.
- Choose fish with the lowest levels of contaminants. These include wild Alaskan salmon (fresh, frozen, or canned), Atlantic mackerel and herring, sardines, sablefish, anchovies, and farmed oysters.
- Avoid farm-raised fish entirely.
- Avoid fish with the highest levels of mercury, including canned albacore, swordfish, tilefish, king mackerel, tuna steaks, and whale.

It takes energy—calories—to absorb, digest, and store proteins, carbohydrates, and fats. Your body uses about twice as many calories to break down protein as to break down fats and carbohydrates, which means that protein helps rev up your metabolic rate.

That said, your body cannot store extra protein for later use, so if you consume more protein than your body needs, you'll store the excess (like any other extra calorie) as sugar and fat.

However, protein is an ally in your weight-loss battle for a couple of reasons. First, protein causes the secretion of glucagon, which tells your body to stop storing fat and to burn it. Second, because protein creates a higher ratio of glucagon to insulin, your blood sugar stays more stable, which helps you stave off crashes and cravings.

This brings up one of the most important advantages of an animal-protein diet versus a vegetarian or vegan diet when it comes to fat loss. It's true that you can get all of the essential amino acids your body needs by eating a combination of grains and legumes, i.e., beans and rice. The individual amino acids will be there, but they come with a high carb load, and thus a high insulin surge—and what's worse, they do not trigger glucagon production. The higher glucagon-to-insulin ratio associated with an animal-protein diet is key for fat loss, sending the message to burn fat, while insulin alone sends the message to store, store, store.

For all the benefits of protein, some varieties are healthier than others. Although most high-protein diets are not picky about the types of protein they allow, this program encourages you to be selective.

For example, compared with grass-fed beef or bison or with fish, conventionally raised red meat contains significantly more saturated fat and fewer superfats like CLA (conjugated linoleic acid) and omega-3 fatty acids (more to come on essential fatty acids and omega-3s). The Optimal proteins on the Ultimate You plan include organically raised, hormone- and antibiotic-free, lean animal proteins such as chicken, turkey, game meat, grass-fed beef and bison, and wild-caught fish.

THE TRUTH ABOUT FAT

For the most part, we've emerged from the fat-phobic culture of the '80s, and nearly everyone now understands that fat is a vital part of a healthy diet. Your body needs all types of dietary fat: saturated, monounsaturated, and polyunsaturated fats (a.k.a. essential fatty acids).

fish oils for fat loss

Fish oils do more than just protect your health. Omega-3 fatty acids are one of the "essential fatty acids" necessary in our diet. They are important nutrients for the heart, brain, skin, and reproductive system—helping you stay lean, pretty, and sexy. Their anti-inflammatory properties also protect you from chronic disease. Because our diets and our food sources are so deficient in these fats, supplementation is a very good idea—especially when it comes to fat loss.

Like hormones, fish oils act as metabolic messengers. They send information deep into your cells, bind receptors on a cell's nucleus, and switch on genes that in turn make more enzymes that burn fat.

Fish oils produce fat loss even in those who don't exercise, studies have shown. However, teaming exercise and fish oils works even better. A study in the *American Journal of Clinical Nutrition* (May 2007) found that people who exercised and supplemented with 6 grams of fish oil per day lost nearly 3½ pounds of body fat in 12 weeks.

Omega-3s are found in other foods besides fish, such as nuts and flaxseed. Although widely prescribed as an omega-3 supplement, flaxseed oil does not contain the forms of omega-3s responsible for fat burning: EPA and DHA. Fish oil does. Your body would have to convert flaxseed oil into EPA and DHA—a slow process, if your body does it at all. In fact, you would need over 10 times the amount of flaxseed oil to get the EPA and DHA found in fish oil. Flax is also easily oxidized, making rancid supplements a huge problem.

That's why we recommend fish oil as the best omega-3 source. For fat loss, take the amount of fish oil used in the study: 6 grams per day, spread throughout the day. Some experts prescribe up to 30 grams per day or more for their overweight patients, but if you take more than 10 grams of fish oil per day for more than 4 months, we recommend that you work with a qualified health-care practitioner who can monitor your essential fatty acid balance. Despite popular belief, you can take too many omega-3s. To learn about choosing a high-quality fish-oil supplement, see page 128.

Note: Fish oils can thin the blood. If you take blood-thinning medications, such as coumadin and aspirin, consult your doctor before you take fish oil. And remember to stop fish-oil supplements 1 week before you undergo a surgical procedure.

- **Monounsaturated fats:** Often dubbed the good fats, monos are important ammunition in weight loss, healthy cholesterol levels, and hunger regulation. Monos are found in nuts, nut butters, avocados, olives, and olive oil.

- **Essential fatty acids (EFAs):** These polyunsaturated fats, a.k.a. essential fats, are found in fatty fish, as well as in some nuts and seeds. They are called essential because your body can't make them—you must get them from food. The main forms of these fats are the omega-6s and the omega-3s. In the simplest terms, omega-6s are "pro-inflammatory," while omega-3s are considered "anti-inflammatory." There are two particular omega-3s: eicosapentaenoic acid (EPA) and docosahexaenoic acid (DHA). They are the building blocks

do you have a d-ficiency?

Vitamin D is crucial in bone and cartilage strength, nervous system health, and immune function. It's also important for weight loss: Because vitamin D improves insulin sensitivity, it helps improve tolerance to carbohydrates.

And yet an estimated 60 percent of Americans are deficient in D, according to a survey by the Centers for Disease Control and Prevention (CDC). Reasons for this national deficit are low-fat diets, poor digestion, and possibly the overuse of sunscreen. Apparently, we've heeded the "use sunscreen" message so well that we're missing out on beneficial vitamin D. Aged skin, darker pigmented skin, and living in northern latitudes all increase the risk of vitamin D deficiency.

You get vitamin D from three sources: sunlight, food, and supplements. Here's how to get more D.

■ Eat more D-rich foods, such as salmon, mackerel, sardines, and tuna. And don't skimp on dietary fat (necessary for vitamin D absorption).

■ Get some sun for 10 minutes, with skin exposed during a time of day when the sun is directly overhead. If you have fair skin, take extra precautions to avoid getting burned, and, of course, no matter what your skin type, avoid getting sunburns.

■ Some experts suspect that the current recommended daily values—200 international units (IU) for adults up to age 50, 400 IU for those ages 51 to 70, and 600 IU for people 71 and older—may be too low. Take a multivitamin with at least 400 IU daily. If your levels are low, you may need up to 5,000 IU daily to replete a serious deficiency—consult with a health-care professional if you suspect a vitamin D deficiency.

■ Have your doctor test your vitamin D levels using the 25-hydroxy vitamin D test—a.k.a. 25(OH)D test. The optimum level is 50 to 80 nanograms per milliliter. Get tested before you begin taking supplements, as it is possible to get too much D.

■ If your test reveals a deficiency, add a supplement. Opt for a product that contains the D_3 form of vitamin D as well as vitamin K (200 mcg of vitamin K per 2,000 IU of vitamin D_3).

for chemicals (called cytokines) that control immune function, blood clotting, and cell growth, as well as components of cell membranes. Omega-3s are plentiful in fish, grass-fed animals, and some nuts. Omega-3s reduce inflammation, which is an important component of the immune response, but in the modern world, inflammation is nearly out of control. EPA and DHA are also key for fat loss.

Omega-6s are found mainly in grains and refined vegetable oils—used in most snack foods, cookies, crackers, and sweets—and are higher in meat of grain-fed animals. Cytokines made from omega-6s tend to increase inflammation, blood clotting, and cell proliferation.

Humans used to consume omega-6 and omega-3 fatty acids in roughly a 2-to-1 ratio. Today, we consume closer to a 24-to-1 ratio! Why? The Westernized junk-food diet is too high in grain-based foods (i.e., breads, pastas, and sugars) and low-quality protein, providing far too many omega-6s and not enough omega-3s. This imbalance may explain the rise of inflammatory conditions such as asthma, heart disease, and some cancers.

On the Ultimate You plan, you'll consume lots of omega-3s in the form of fish, nuts, and grass-fed beef or bison. The plan also recommends a high-quality omega-3 fish-oil supplement (details to come in Phase 1).

- **Saturated fats:** Saturated fats are found in animal proteins, eggs and dairy, and coconut oil and coconut milk. Eaten in sensible amounts, saturated fat isn't your body's enemy. In fact, this fat is important for your brain, hormones, and cell membranes. That said, it's wise to monitor your intake of foods higher in saturated fat because this type of fat is the hardest to burn as energy.

And there are a few uniquely healthy saturated fats. First, the medium-chain triglycerides in coconut oil and coconut milk provide incredibly clean-burning fuel. Next, butter contains the short-chain fatty acids important for fueling the healthy bacteria in the gut.

A good rule of thumb: Consume most of your dietary fat as nuts, olives, olive oil, coconut oil, avocados, and cold-water fish (from both food and supplements) and the remainder from saturated animal fat, such as grass-fed animals, free-range poultry, and organic eggs. Don't sweat the calculations:

drink more water, lose more fat

To burn fat, your cells need to be well hydrated—swollen up like tiny water balloons. When full of water, they're able to keep their pH in range. At a proper pH, enzymes, which are a cell's machinery, can work properly. Some of that work is to burn fat and make proteins. And because thirst can be mistaken as hunger, being well hydrated can make it easier for you to stick to your eating plan.

How can you tell if you're dehydrated? One undeniable sign: thirst. You may also get more headaches, feel tired, get more easily pooped than usual during workouts, or develop constipation or dry skin. You might also catch more colds and flu bugs, or allergies and joint pain may worsen.

The advice to drink eight 8-ounce glasses of water a day is outdated. Instead, multiply your weight in pounds by 0.5 and 0.7. The numbers generated are the range, in ounces, of filtered water you should drink each day.

Don't drink anywhere near that amount? No need to start chugging it down. Instead, gradually increase your intake over a 4-week period. When you start, you'll be thirstier and pay more visits to the ladies' room, but you'll adjust.

Other water-y advice:

- Drink filtered water whenever possible to avoid the microbial contaminants, chlorine, fluorine, and heavy metals common in tap water.

- Avoid bottled water as much as possible. Plastic water bottles can leach estrogenic chemicals.

- Before you give in to a craving, drink a glass of water instead.

- If you exercise or perform intense physical activity in hot weather, your body's need for water and electrolytes increases. Pass up the sugary sports drinks and opt instead for coconut water or Hardware's Ultimate Electrolytes (1 packet 1 or 2 times daily; avoid if you have heart or kidney problems or high blood pressure).

- If you get bored with plain water, treat yourself to sparkling water with a twist of lemon or lime or to a no-sugar designer water, such as Hint Water or Ayala's Herbal Water. You can also use the recipes below to mix up your own fancy H_2O.

- **Sweet Water:** Add ½ teaspoon (more or less to taste) Truvia sweetener to cherry or orange sparkling water.

- **Lemon Fizz:** Add ½ teaspoon (more or less to taste) Truvia sweetener and 1 teaspoon lemon juice to lemon-lime sparkling water.

- **Chocolate Raspberry or Vanilla Stevia Sipper:** Add 5 drops SweetLeaf brand liquid stevia Chocolate Raspberry flavor to raspberry sparkling water, or add 5 drops of French Vanilla to plain sparkling water.

If you stick to the recommended lean proteins and recommended fats, you'll do fine.

THE ULTIMATE YOU PLAN: SIMPLE AND EFFECTIVE

Like your workouts, your nutrition plan is laid out for you in four easy-to-follow phases. Your food choices are divided into two groups.

Optimal choices include the leanest proteins; the healthiest, easiest-to-burn fats; high-fiber, plant-based starchy carbs; and lots of nutritious nonstarchy vegetables.

Allowable choices include proteins that are slightly more processed, low-fat dairy products, and a few grain-based but still high-fiber starchy carbs. These will give you more options as you utilize the plan.

In Phase 1, you can eat from either group. In Phases 2 through 4, we strongly encourage you to stick to the Optimal choices for better results.

The nutrition program itself is pretty simple—stick to your Optimal and Allowable choices, and you should have the hang of it after just a few days. Commit these seven habits to memory, practice them daily, and before long, you'll see your Ultimate You begin to take shape.

1. Eat breakfast every day; make sure it contains both protein and vegetables.
2. Eat at least 5 to 6 servings of vegetables per day (1 cup = 1 serving).
3. Eat high-quality lean protein—4 to 6 ounces at a meal, and 2 to 3 ounces per snack.
4. Drink 3 to 4 liters of filtered water each day.
5. Opt for organic fruits and vegetables and organic, hormone-free meat, poultry, and fish whenever you can.
6. Stick to the plan 90 percent of the time; enjoy 1 splurge meal per week.
7. Stay focused on success. Reaffirm your goals at least once daily, more often if the going gets tough.

THE ULTIMATE YOU FOODS LIST

We've organized foods into Allowable/Optimal/Avoid lists, then further divided them into carbs, proteins, and fats. We'll give you more specific instructions as you move through

coffee conundrum

Keep your morning cup of coffee—it's loaded with antioxidants and you'll lose more weight when hopped up on caffeine. No, wait—all that caffeine might cause diabetes and is bad for weight loss. What should you do? Here's what you really need to know:

- Caffeine appears to acutely lower one's insulin sensitivity, but the effect is not chronic; in healthy individuals, coffee drinking does not lead to diabetes.

- Avoid drinking it with starches (Optimal or Allowable, and skip the muffin for sure at your coffee break). If you have insulin resistance, diabetes, or are not following a lower-carb diet, caffeine can make insulin matters worse. One way to mitigate this negative insulin response is to add ¼ teaspoon cinnamon to your cup of joe.

- Raising epinephrine is one mechanism by which caffeine perks you up. A preworkout cup of coffee or tea will allow you to perform better, exercise harder, and burn more fat at the gym. Avoid post-workout caffeine to avoid thwarting the effects of your Recovery Shake. And if you have anxiety, insomnia, or are at all aggravated from caffeine, it's wise to steer clear of coffee and caffeinated beverages in general.

- The fat in cream or half-and-half slows the release of caffeine into your system, making it a better fat burner. But keep portions to one tablespoon or less so as not to pile on the calories and saturated fat.

- Caffeine appears to be less of a diuretic than once thought—meaning it isn't as significant of a factor in dehydration.

- Because caffeine is metabolized by the liver by the same enzymes that clear out estrogen, coffee in an estrogen-dominant woman can make matters worse and hinder fat loss.

the phases, but here's a quick rundown of how it works: It's easy! You can choose from Optimal or Allowed. If you want to lose fat more quickly, stick to the Optimal list.

Ultimate You Carbohydrates

OPTIMAL CARBS

Eat nonstarchy vegetables raw, steamed, sautéed, stir-fried, or roasted at every meal. Try to always choose one green veggie and one that's brightly colored (i.e., red, yellow, orange, purple).

Eat high-fiber fruit or a high-fiber starch in the recommended amounts at each meal, if desired. In Phase 2, you will be given modified options for carb intake.

NONSTARCHY VEGETABLES

You may have unlimited amounts of these; aim for a minimum of 5 servings per day.

- Artichokes
- Arugula
- Asparagus
- Bamboo shoots
- Bean sprouts
- Beet greens
- Bell peppers
- Broccoli
- Carrots
- Cauliflower
- Celery
- Chayote fruit
- Chicory
- Chives
- Collard greens
- Coriander leaf
- Cucumber
- Dandelion greens
- Eggplant
- Endive
- Fava beans
- Fennel
- Green beans
- Hearts of palm
- Jicama (raw)

- Jalapeño or any other hot chile peppers (poblano, Anaheim, ancho chile, etc.)
- Kale
- Kohlrabi
- Lettuce (any variety: mixed greens, romaine, green or red leaf, butter, etc.)
- Mushrooms
- Mustard greens
- Onions
- Parsley
- Radicchio
- Radishes
- Snap beans
- Snow peas
- Shallots
- Spaghetti squash
- Spinach
- Summer squash (i.e., zucchini)
- Swiss chard
- Tomatoes
- Turnip greens
- Watercress
- Fresh herbs: basil, cilantro, mint, rosemary, thyme, etc. (These make excellent, flavorful, and healthy additions to salads—delicious!)

HIGH-FIBER/LOWER-SUGAR FRUITS

Examples of serving sizes: ½ cup berries, 1 medium apple or pear.

- Apples (any variety)

- Berries (blackberries, blueberries, raspberries, etc.)

- Cherries (any variety)

- Pears (any variety)

HIGH-FIBER STARCHES

Stick to 4 to 6 bites or ⅓- to ½-cup servings.

- Beans/legumes (azuki, black beans, cannellini beans, garbanzo beans, kidney beans, etc.)

- Sweet potatoes, yams, or pumpkin

- Winter squashes

ALLOWABLE CARBS

HIGH-FIBER GRAIN-BASED STARCHES

Limit these to the servings listed.

- Steel-cut oats or Irish oatmeal (⅓ to ½ cup or 4 to 6 bites)

- Old-fashioned whole, rolled oats (⅓ to ½ cup or 4 to 6 bites)

- Oat bran (⅓ to ½ cup or 4 to 6 bites)

- High-fiber hemp bread (limit to 1 slice per meal or 4 to 6 bites)

- Sprouted-grain breads, such as Ezekial 4:9 (limit to 1 slice per meal or 4 to 6 bites)

- Sprouted-grain English-style muffins or bagels (½ muffin or bagel)

- Other sprouted-grain products, such as wraps or tortillas (1 tortilla or wrap)

- GG Crispbread (highest fiber/best choice), FiberRich crackers, or Wasa or Ryvita crispbread (2 crackers)

- Quinoa (⅓ to ½ cup or 4 to 6 bites)

MODERATE-FIBER/MODERATE-SUGAR FRUITS

Limit these to 2 or 3 times per week.

- Apricots (fresh)
- Grapefruit
- Kiwifruit
- Melon (honeydew, cantaloupe, etc.)
- Nectarines
- Oranges
- Passion fruit
- Peaches
- Persimmons
- Pitted prunes
- Plums
- Pomegranates
- Tangerines

LOWER-FIBER/HIGHER-SUGAR FRUITS

These are only allowed 2 hours or less after a workout.

- Bananas
- Grapes
- Mangoes
- Papayas
- Pineapple
- Watermelon

STARCHES, CARBS, AND SUGARS TO AVOID

Avoid these foods unless they're part of your cheat meal. If they are, enjoy them fully!

- Regular breads, including whole grain breads—only hemp or sprouted-grain breads are allowed
- Any baked goods, including doughnuts, pastries, muffins, cookies, cakes, pies, and other desserts
- White potatoes
- Dry cereals (even high-protein or sprouted-grain varieties)
- Sugar in all its forms: table sugar, candy, soda, anything containing high-fructose corn syrup, organic sugar, brown sugar, evaporated cane juice, agave, molasses, maple syrup, date sugar, fruit juice concentrate, raw sugar, sucanat, and turbinado sugar (honey will have a limited role in your plan; more on that in Chapter 7 and with the recipe for your Recovery Shake on page 37)

- Artificial sweeteners and/or any product that contains them: aspartame, sucralose, acesulfame K, and saccharin (refer to page 91 for more on sweeteners)

- Dried fruit, which is higher in sugar because its water content has been sapped out so the water can't interact with the fiber; what's more, dried fruit is often covered in sugar and oil (e.g., dried cranberries are typically coated in sunflower oil and sugar); you may occasionally sprinkle dried fruit over a salad or drop a dried apricot into a cup of hot green tea to add sweetness and a delicious fruit flavor, but for the most part stick with fresh fruit

- Sugar-laden condiments: barbecue sauce, ketchup, relish (read labels and refer to page 264)

- Energy bars and most protein bars (see page 93 for Allowed bars)

- Ice cream (including fat-free products like frozen-fruit bars, gelato, frozen yogurt, and rice- or soy-based frozen desserts)

- Popcorn, chips, and pretzels (including sweet potato or veggie chips)

Ultimate You Proteins

OPTIMAL PROTEINS

These foods are ideal based on fat content and quality; ideal serving size is 4 to 6 ounces.

- Grass-fed buffalo or bison
- Grass-fed beef
- Game (venison, elk, boar, etc.)
- Lean chicken breast/ground chicken breast
- Turkey breast/ground white-meat turkey
- Cornish game hens
- Ostrich
- Pheasant
- Organic, omega-3, cage-free eggs

- Organic egg whites (read labels and avoid those with added sugar or colors; while egg whites are a very low-fat protein option, we feel that eating them can cheat you out of some valuable nutrients—if you prefer egg whites, try to include at least 1 whole egg in your scramble or omelet)
- Wild salmon (fresh or canned)
- Shellfish (shrimp, crab, scallops, lobster, etc.)
- Halibut

OPTIMAL PROTEINS CONTINUED

- Cod
- Atlantic mackerel
- Herring
- Flounder
- Bass
- Grouper
- Mahi-mahi
- Perch
- Pike
- Pollack (often available as "fake crab" or "fake lobster" meat; good low-fat protein, but substitute products often have added sugar, so read labels)
- Trout
- Rockfish (a.k.a. ocean perch)
- Orange roughy
- Sardines
- Snapper
- Tilapia
- Sole
- Turbot
- Whey protein (see recommended brands on page 37)
- Natural jerky: Ostrich, turkey, and beef jerky is available at many health-food stores and makes a great snack. However, avoid jerky made from tempeh or soy.

ALLOWABLE PROTEINS

Try to choose fresh or frozen meats. If you go for more processed proteins, read labels and avoid brands made with added sugar, nitrates, excess sodium, chemical preservatives, or artificial colors/dyes. Applegate Farms has some good uncured, nitrate-free, and no-hormone options. All dairy products should be low-fat, organic, and hormone free.

- Lean red meats (not grass-fed; limit to 2 or 3 times per week), including: tenderloin, filet mignon, flank steak, sirloin, round steak, and roast beef
- Pork (boiled lean ham, loin chop, or pork tenderloin)
- Lamb (limit to once a week—higher saturated fat)
- Smoked or canned salmon or canned smoked trout
- Low-fat cottage cheese
- Low-fat feta/goat cheese
- Low-fat ricotta cheese
- Light Jarlsberg Swiss
- Parmesan
- Low-fat yogurt (Greek yogurt is higher in protein, not to mention thick and delicious!)

PROTEINS TO AVOID

Avoid these foods as much as possible.

- Corned beef
- Hot dogs (even chicken or turkey varieties)
- Lunch meat (except for organic, nitrate-free versions, such as Applegate Farms)
- Pastrami
- Prosciutto

Ultimate You Fats

OPTIMAL FATS

All food items containing fat should be organic.

- Raw nuts and seeds: almonds, Brazil nuts, cashews, hazelnuts, peanuts, pecans, pine nuts, pistachios, walnuts, pumpkin seeds, sunflower seeds, etc.
- Natural nut butters (almond, cashew, peanut, etc): Be sure to read labels and opt for brands without added sugar or salt.
- Freshly ground flaxseed meal (not flax oil or preground flaxseed): Flaxseed can help with hormone balance due to its lignan content; be sure to get whole seeds, keep them refrigerated, and grind as needed in a coffee grinder. Or try this soaking technique: Place 1 tablespoon flaxseed in a small glass, cover with water, and let sit overnight so they will be a little "slippery" and soft come morning, then drink them down like a "shot" or add to a protein shake or a serving of high-fiber starch, such as oat bran or sweet potato.
- Olive oil: organic, first cold press, in a dark bottle (darker glass offers better protection from oxidation), or as a spray
- Olives (fresh, canned, or jarred)
- Avocado and guacamole
- Coconut milk and coconut oil: Coconut is a very stable and healthy saturated fat, making it one of the best cooking oils—its medium-chain triglycerides make great fuel. Use it for sautés or stir-fries, or add 1 tablespoon to a protein shake or

high-fiber starch like oat bran or sweet potato or even as a salad dressing for a
light coconut flavor. (Don't worry if it appears a little waxy—it's solid at room
temperature.)

- Walnut oil (as salad dressing, not for cooking)
- Avocado oil (as salad dressing, not for cooking)
- Macadamia nut oil (as salad dressing or for cooking)

ALLOWABLE FATS

Due to their higher saturated-fat content, limit these foods to 2 to 3 servings per week
during Phases 1 and 2.

- Macadamia nuts
- Organic butter

FATS TO AVOID

- Commercially prepared salad dressings: They're often loaded with sugar
  (particularly low-fat varieties) and usually contain "bad fats" and preservatives;
  dress your salads with oil and vinegar (using olive, avocado, macadamia, or
  walnut oil) or lemon juice and seasonings.
- Butter spray substitutes
- Vegetable-oil spreads and margarine
- All trans fats, hydrogenated fats, lard, and fried foods
- Corn, safflower, sunflower, and peanut oils
- Coffee creamers: If you lighten your coffee or tea, try using half-and-half
  or cream—although high in saturated fat, the amount used is low, and the
  fat will help buffer a big caffeine dose, slowing the rate of absorption into the
  bloodstream. If you prefer flavored coffee, add 5 drops of flavored liquid stevia
  (such as SweetLeaf Vanilla Cream or Chocolate Raspberry) instead.
- Conventional mayonnaise (opt for olive oil– or nut oil–based mayo)

Miscellaneous Allowed Foods

- Organic cream or organic half-and-half: fine in your coffee or tea

- Organic coffee: Try to limit coffee consumption to 1 cup per day (if you drink it).

- Organic black, green, and herbal teas: The Numi brand has a great selection.

- Garlic: one of the healthiest foods on the planet; use fresh and dried as much as possible

- Gingerroot

- Dry spices: Herbs and spices will help you manage your salt intake as they add zest to your meals; many also boast natural antibiotic, antiviral, and anti-inflammatory properties (turmeric and cayenne pepper, in particular, are well-documented anti-inflammatories). Here are some of the standouts, with some suggestions for use.

  - *Cinnamon* helps manage blood sugar; add to coffee, yogurt, oats, sweet potato, or a protein shake.

  - *Dill* is an excellent addition to a veggie egg scramble; or mix it with fat-free yogurt and add a dollop to salmon.

  - *Paprika* is excellent sprinkled on eggs or fish; blend with a dollop of fat-free yogurt and use as a condiment.

  - *Chipotle* pepper has a smoky-sweet flavor that adds a yummy zing to chicken, eggs, and veggies.

  - *Sea salt* is a better option than table salt.

- Natural vanilla extract: Add to protein shakes or yogurt if desired, and sweeten with stevia or xylitol. To nip a craving or as a natural treatment for insomnia, add to unsweetened almond milk with a pinch of stevia or xylitol, 1 teaspoon nutmeg (a natural sedative), and ½ teaspoon cinnamon and serve warm.

- Organic unsweetened cocoa powder: Add a tablespoon to your Recovery Shake to boost its antioxidant capacity, or try a cup of our Ultimate You Cocoa (recipe on page 167).

- Unsweetened shredded coconut

- Marinara or other tomato sauce: 1 serving equals ½ cup; choose a brand that contains 5 grams of carbs or less, and check labels for added sugar

- Sweeteners: Truvia (brand name of sweetener that contains erythritol and stevia), stevia, and xylitol

- Tahini (sesame-seed paste)

- Mustard (natural, no artificial colors or sugar added)

- Hot sauces: Most are simple blends of peppers, vinegar, and salt, but read labels for added sugar; there are lots of options—Louisiana style, Mexican, South American, etc.

- Salsa (no sugar added)

- Vinegars: balsamic, white balsamic, white wine, red wine, rice, plum, apple cider, etc.; experiment with flavored vinegars for more exciting salads (again, watch for added sugar)

- Worcestershire sauce

- Organic lemon and lime juice: Use with oil for salad dressings or add to water or sparkling water.

- Unsweetened dairy substitutes, such as almond milk or So Delicious brand coconut milk

CHAPTER 7

Preparing for the Ultimate You

IT'S A CLICHÉ, BUT THE old saying "Failure to plan is planning to fail" is absolutely true. The biggest excuse we hear from clients struggling to make a nutrition or exercise plan work is lack of time. You will never be given time to get fit and healthy. You have to make time.

One way to make time in the future is to spend a little time now preparing your kitchen, your office, and your lifestyle for success on the Ultimate You plan. Until you do, you will inevitably struggle with meal timing, getting caught without a suitable snack, running out of cooked protein choices, and a myriad of other common but preventable challenges.

> You will never be given time to get fit and healthy. You have to make time.

Once you have all the necessary items and learn how to navigate the grocery store, how to cook and plan ahead, and how to order out, you will not find yourself at the mercy of time. Preparing for the Ultimate You means learning a few new tricks, dismantling some big weight-loss myths, and changing your mind about priorities and discipline.

By the end of this chapter, you'll learn how to fend off cravings, monitor your progress, and self-correct when you get off track. In short, you'll be raring to go at the start of Phase 1. Next comes creating the Ultimate You—so get ready!

MAKE OVER YOUR KITCHEN

Now's the time to do some quick kitchen cleanup and toss out foods and products that do not support your Ultimate You. This decreases the temptation to stray from your nutrition program and creates space for the new healthy foods in your kitchen.

If any of the foods below lurk in your fridge, freezer, or pantry, donate them where possible, or throw them out. It may be tough to do this, but believe us, it will be worth it in the end—losing body fat is worth more than whatever you paid for them!

- Frozen dinners (including low-calorie or "diet" brands)
- Table sugar (white, refined sugar)
- Regular salt (replace with sea salt)
- Any "regular" breads or baked goods (including any bread other than sprouted or high-protein hemp bread, pastries, muffins, etc.)
- Any dry or fresh pasta
- Sweeteners other than xylitol, stevia, erythritol (under several brand names, including Truvia or Zerose), and honey (for your post-workout shakes in Phases 2 through 4)
- Sugar-laden condiments, including ketchup, barbecue sauce, teriyaki sauce, and many prepared salad dressings (read labels)
- Cereals (with the exception of whole rolled oats, steel-cut oats, or oat bran)

gear up for healthy cooking

You probably already have a cutting board, knife, and a few pots and pans. But arm yourself with the items below, too. They'll help make this plan a breeze.

- Glass Pyrex dishes to store and pack take-along meals—glass is safe to reheat food in, while plastics, which leach estrogenic compounds, are not

- A blender to whip up protein shakes at home and a hard plastic (PCB-free) or glass shaker bottle to make them on the go
- A colander in which to wash greens and other produce
- A salad spinner and a small food processor

- Any peanut or other nut butter that is not natural or contains added sugar

- Any cooking oils other than coconut, olive, or macadamia nut

- Any animal proteins that are not organic, free-range, antibiotic, and hormone free; or farm-raised fish

- "Healthy junk food" such as soy chips, gluten-/wheat-free cookies, or the like. Remember, just because you bought it at a health-food store doesn't mean it's good for you or your weight loss.

GET YOUR GROCERIES

Most supermarkets are laid out with produce, dairy, and meat products along the outside of the store, with processed foods in the center aisles. As you shop, you will spend most of your time on the periphery of the store, then hit a few of the inner aisles for miscellaneous items. Here's how to navigate the perimeter of the supermarket first. That's where you'll find your two most important food groups: produce and proteins.

> Your two most important food groups: produce and proteins

Produce

Pile your cart high with luscious leaves and brightly colored fruits and veggies. Don't know what to choose? Select at least three greens (e.g., lettuce, spinach, broccoli, kale, etc.) and at least three brightly colored veggies (e.g., tomato, yellow bell pepper, purple onion, etc). Purchase high-fiber fruits like berries, apples, and pears, too.

Each time you shop, try a new fruit or veggie. You'll avoid boredom and get a full range of phytonutrients and antioxidants.

Opt for organic produce as much as possible. If you have to make a choice, consider these guidelines: If you eat the skin (for example, on apples), opt for organic. If it is a hearty plant that you can wash thoroughly (e.g., tough kale leaves versus more flimsy lettuce), you can more safely skimp on not going organic.

If you're worried that you've loaded up on fresh produce that will just rot in the fridge, follow this simple guideline: Eat flimsy greens—such as lettuce, fresh herbs, and spinach—within the first few days of purchase. The heartier kale, chard, bok choy, broccoli, zucchini, cucumber, celery, and asparagus will last for a week or longer.

simple veggie wash

Wash all produce, even organic produce. Besides pesticides, you're still dealing with dirt, the occasional insect, and all the dirty hands that have touched your apple as they sifted through the bin. There are several commercially available natural veggie washes, but here's an inexpensive and easy-to-make alternative.

1 part distilled white vinegar

3 parts plain filtered water

Combine the above in a spray bottle and mist over produce. Then rinse with cool water, let drain, prep, and store in the fridge. This mixture keeps for several months.

For example, if you buy a bag of mixed greens, a head of broccoli, a bunch of red Swiss chard, and a plastic clamshell of spinach, you would first eat the mixed greens and half of the spinach as salads. The next day, sauté the rest of the spinach or eat as another salad. Later that week, steam or stir-fry the broccoli and the Swiss chard.

Eat most other veggies within 2 weeks. These include bell peppers and tomatoes, which, uncut, last about that long. When these veggies start to "turn" and look less than desirable for a salad, stir-fry them or add to scrambled eggs or an omelet.

Proteins

Although you'll spend more, high-quality, lean proteins—preferably organic—are essential to your fat loss. Look for the following wording on protein labels.

- *Chicken/turkey*: hormone free, antibiotic free, free range, organic; available as breasts, cutlets, and ground (opt for ground white over ground dark)

- *Lean beef/buffalo/bison*: hormone free, grass fed, grass finished; available as steaks and ground; other cuts available on occasion

- *Fish*: Look for wild fish (steer clear of farm raised)—previously frozen is fine; avoid swordfish, tilefish, king mackerel, tuna steaks, and whale, as they have the highest mercury levels.

- *Eggs*: organic, cage-free, high omega-3 eggs (ideal) or organic cage-free eggs; for cartons of organic egg whites, read labels and avoid artificial colors and added sugar

- *Dairy*: hormone and antibiotic free, rBGH free, organic; available as organic yogurt, half-and-half, milk, and cheese

An important point: When protein is labeled "organic," it means the animals were fed organic feed. However, it does not necessarily mean they were hormone or antibiotic free, and it definitely does not mean "free range" or "grass fed."

Your supermarket may not carry all of these protein options. If that's the case, make the best choices you can as often as you can. For example, you might look for organic meats and dairy at a local farmers' market. If you can't find grass-fed, grass-finished beef or bison locally, consider having it shipped to you. A great online resource is www.grasslandbeef.com.

NAVIGATE THE AISLES

At this point, your cart will be nearly full with tasty, lean cuts of protein and beautiful fresh veggies and fruit. Now round out your meals with the items below.

SPICES: Spices add pizzazz to healthy meals. As a bonus, they're chock-full of antioxidants, natural antimicrobials, and natural anti-inflammatories.

Some common favorites are sea salt, cracked black pepper, crushed red pepper flakes, Italian seasoning, cinnamon, crushed garlic, and ginger. But we encourage you to branch out and experiment.

To *really* spice things up, add hot sauces, spicy or regular mustards (opt for no artificial dyes or colors and no sugar), jars or cans of olives, jarred or fresh salsas, or a variety of flavored vinegars to use on salads and vegetables.

COOKING OILS: Again, spend a bit more—your body and health will thank you. Most toxins, hormones, and problematic chemicals are fat soluble, so opt for organic oils, if available.

time-savers

Instead of unloading grocery bags right into the fridge, deal with your produce first—you'll be more likely to use it. These quick tips can help.

- Wash and spin your lettuce to keep it crisp and help it last longer. Keep it in the salad spinner and store in the fridge.

- Cut up veggies (cucumbers, radishes, peppers, celery, carrots, mushrooms) and place them in Pyrex bowls, then refrigerate. It's fine to buy prewashed, precut veggies. They're more expensive and won't last as long, but if you're more likely to use them, go for it.

- While you wash and chop, try this supereasy recipe: Preheat the oven to 350°F. Place 4 chicken breasts in a glass baking dish and pour 1 cup of chicken broth over them. Add a dash of sea salt, pepper, garlic powder, and Italian seasoning (or your favorite seasonings), then pop in the oven. Bake 30 minutes or until done.

The must-haves: organic coconut oil (in a jar, solid at room temperature, looks like wax), olive oil (organic, first cold-pressed in a dark glass bottle to discourage oxidation), and macadamia nut oil. This trio offers variety and ensures that you cook with oils that won't be damaged by heat. Both coconut oil and macadamia nut oil have high smoking points and can handle hotter temperatures; olive oil stands up to moderate heat. For salad dressings, use olive oil or try a light nut oil—like walnut or sesame (not to be used for cooking).

CENTER-AISLE ALLOWABLES: A few packaged items can help you cook more creatively and expand your meal options. These include high-fiber carbs like canned or dry beans; organic canned pumpkin; organic coconut milk; jarred marinara sauce (no sugar added) or canned tomatoes and tomato sauce to make your own sauce; and quick, healthy proteins such as canned tuna, sardines, and salmon. If you like olives, add a jar to your cart—olives can help nip a craving for salty snacks like potato

how to *really* read a label

Calories, grams of protein, total cholesterol—what do the numbers on nutrition labels really tell you? While you'll eat few packaged foods on this plan, it's good to know how to decipher a label. Here's what to look for.

■ **Scan for portion size.** Portion sizes listed on labels—on both foods and beverages—can be deceiving. What you assume is one serving may be two or even three. Take a closer look.

■ **Peruse for partially hydrogenated oils.** If you find them on the label, place the product back on the shelf.

■ **Suss out hidden sources of sugar.** Just a few of the words you don't want to see: *fructose, dextrose, cane juice, high-fructose corn syrup,* and *fruit juice.*

■ **Use this handy "carb formula."** Typically, packaged foods contain significant amounts of carbohydrates. Use this formula to keep on track.

1. Add the fiber and protein grams.

2. Subtract that number from the total number of carbs.

3. Consider your result. If the number is:

 ■ **Greater than 10:** The food is too high in carbs relative to fiber and protein.

 ■ **Between 5 and 10:** The food is acceptable.

 ■ **5 or less:** The food fits the bill for fat loss.

For more information on label lingo, see the Appendix (page 263).

chips. Note: The lining of most cans contains problematic plastics that can leach endocrine disruptors, so opt for glass jars whenever possible or buy certain items dry, such as beans.

Other middle-aisle Allowable foods include:

- Whole rolled oats, steel-cut oats, and oat bran

- High-fiber crackers, such as GG Crispbread, FiberRich, Wasa, and Ryvita—they're yummy, and Allowable, crunchy carbs

- Raw nuts and/or natural nut butters (opt for organic, no-sugar varieties); try almond butter or cashew butter—they're delicious

- Organic, unsweetened vanilla or chocolate almond milk (found unrefrigerated, in boxes); use in coffee, as a dairy substitute in cooking, or to thicken up a protein smoothie

One last stop: the frozen section. Keep flash-frozen cut veggies on hand for days when you are out of fresh produce, and make Recovery Shakes with frozen berries and cherries. (Fun fact: The antioxidants in frozen berries, such as blueberries, are more available to your body than those in fresh berries.) The frozen-foods section also features sprouted-grain products and hemp bread and—on occasion—frozen salmon burgers or bison burgers.

GET SWEETENER SAVVY

The diet world is filled with mysterious sugar substitutions and the health world with so-called natural sweeteners. Most people experience *fewer* sweet cravings when they stop using sweeteners.

If you are going to sweeten, use sugar alcohols or stevia, a natural sugar. From the plant *Stevia rebaudinana*, called sweet leaf, it is completely natural, is 300 times sweeter than sugar (a little goes a long way!), does not aggravate insulin, and has been designated GRAS (generally regarded as safe) by the FDA—although it's been used safely for decades in Asia. It has a slightly bitter aftertaste, so if you dislike the taste of artificial sweeteners like aspartame, then stick with the sugar alcohols, such as xylitol and erythritol.

Still, it's good to know about all sweeteners, whether they come in a pink packet or in your salad dressing. They fall into three general categories: sugar alcohols (the Good), natural sugars (the Iffy), and chemical sweeteners (the Bad).

The Good: Sugar Alcohols

Found in many low-carb or sugar-free products, these sweeteners have little or no effect on insulin and are from natural sources. While digestive disruption is not unheard of, if you incorporate them slowly into your diet, you'll most likely adapt without issue.

- **Xylitol:** Derived from birch-tree bark and corn husks to make a sweetener that is typically used 1:1 as a substitute for sugar, xylitol (naturally found in fruit) is great on insulin and also slows stomach emptying, helping you feel full quicker. It also helps prevent dental cavities and sinus and middle-ear infections. Use this sweetener as part of your weight loss plan, chew xylitol gum to prevent cavities, and have xylitol nasal spray on hand for sinus infections. Available at www.bodybyhardware. com and as XyloSweet online and in health-food stores (www.xlear.com). (Watch for the addition of silica to some crystalline xylitol products.)

- **Erythritol:** Also found in fruit (although only in small concentrations), erythritol is about 70 percent as sweet as regular sugar. Another no-insulin-response sweetener boasting the ability to support healthy bacteria in our intestines, erythritol is sold under several brand names, including Zerose, Sweet Simplicity, and Truvia (in combination with stevia), and is available in health-food stores.

- **Malitol and sorbitol:** Found in many sugar-free products, malitol and sorbitol are about 80 and 60 percent, respectively, as sweet as sugar. These two cause the most digestive disturbance (bloating and laxative action), so go slow.

The Iffy: Natural Sugars

Health food stores are teeming with so-called healthy sugar: evaporated cane juice, molasses, maple syrup, barley malt, malt syrup, fructose, crystalline fructose, date sugar, fruit juice concentrate, brown sugar, raw sugar, sucanat, turbinado sugar, honey, and agave syrup. Although touted as healthy alternatives, when it comes to insulin, they behave almost just like regular sugar, so they are bad news for fat loss. However, two of these sweeteners, honey and agave, deserve a closer look.

- **Honey:** Honey is 30 percent fructose and 50 percent glucose (white sugar is 50 percent glucose and 50 percent fructose). Use honey only after a workout for fat loss.

Its insulin response is ideal post-workout—just the right amount to lower stress hormones. So consider using 1 teaspoon in your Recovery Shake (recipe on page 37).

- **Agave:** With its low glycemic index (GI score), agave has received a lot of attention as a healthy sugar alternative. It has a low GI because it is nearly all fructose (70 to 90 percent), and GI deals only with glucose loads in the blood, not fructose levels. The very high fructose content makes it very similar to a decidedly unhealthy sweetener: high-fructose corn syrup (HFCS). A large amount of fructose is a problem because it doesn't require insulin (as glucose does), which bypasses a key regulatory step in blood sugar levels and control. Fructose in high amounts (beyond typical fruit consumption) is well documented to worsen insulin resistance, cause free radical damage (i.e., oxidation), and raise cholesterol and triglyceride levels.

The Bad: Chemical Sweeteners

In many "diet" foods, from sodas to Jell-O, the biggies are acesulfame, saccharin (Sweet'N Low), aspartame (Equal, Nutrasweet), and sucralose (Splenda). Acesulfame is terribly lacking in safety research. Both saccharin and aspartame have at least some research linking them to cancer.

One of the biggest problems with aspartame is its potent neurostimulant properties, as it's made from aspartic acid and phenylalanine. Its combination with caffeine in most diet sodas makes it a tough habit to kick and causes withdrawal symptoms such as headaches, nausea, and irritation.

Finally, there's Splenda (a.k.a. sucralose), whose makers tout as "natural" since it's derived from sugar and cite hundreds of studies that show its safety. However, the majority of these

---

raise the bar!

Frankly, we don't recommend most brands of protein bars typically sold in grocery or convenience stores. They tend to contain low-quality proteins such as soy and are too high in calories and carbs (unless they are the low-carb variety) to work well on a fat-loss program.

That said, some low-carb bars have a couple of advantages. If you crave something sweet, they can help you avoid a cookie binge. You can tuck them in your purse or stash them in your car, which can mean the difference between going hungry or going off plan.

The trick is to select bars that meet some rather lofty criteria: They must be low in calories and carbs, made with high-quality whey or rice protein, and taste good. There aren't many that fit that bill, but here are several recommendations.

- Ultimate You Lean Bars (Hardware)

- Biogenesis Low Carb or Ultra Low Carb Bars (Biogenesis)

- Primal Bars (Poliquin Performance)

- PaleoBar (Designs for Health)

While you shouldn't routinely replace meals with bars, it's better to have a bar than miss a meal. It's also best to limit yourself to one bar per day. Enjoy one bar as a snack, or eat half a bar after lunch and the other half after dinner as an on-plan "dessert."

studies were performed on rats, and the few human trials focused on investigating dental cavities, not overall health. And probably most concerning is the fact that sucralose is a chlorinated sugar molecule—a chemical never before seen by nature and something your body can't metabolize. Worse, its close chemical resemblance to a common pesticide warrants caution.

SUPPLEMENT YOUR NUTRITION PLAN

Nutritional supplements are just that—supplemental to a solid nutrition and exercise regimen. But because we overfarm our soil, irradiate our crops, and subject ourselves to incredible stresses, our bodies need extra support from supplements—and that's even if we eat a high-plant diet.

Include at least two and maybe three basic supplements to support your food plan and bolster your overall health and fat loss. Supplements that will support your efforts during each stage of this program are laid out for you phase by phase.

It can be daunting to stand among the rows and rows of vitamins in your health food store—how to choose? If you're like most women, you choose the least expensive version. All supplements are created equal, right? Unfortunately, they're not.

There is little regulation of the nutritional supplement industry—in terms of quality and results, supplements run the gamut from excellent to garbage. Among the issues are "absorption" and "bioavailability" (your body's ability to actually use the nutrients in the capsule); microbial contamination (i.e., bacteria or fungus); unnecessary fillers, artificial colors, and chemical solvents; and accuracy in labeling. Sadly, without regulation, you don't know if what's on the label is what's in the bottle, and many products do not contain a meaningful amount of a nutrient to give you the results you take them for.

While the vast majority are not harmful, they can be less than efficacious. However, there are a handful of supplements (fish oil and vitamin E are good examples) that when of low quality are not only ineffective but could harm your health.

Sidestep Subpar Supplements

We've taken great care to create a line of supplements that meet an extremely high standard of purity and efficacy in order to make it easy for you to follow the recommended protocols in this book. To purchase any supplement from the Hardware line, please visit www.bodybyhardware.com. Within the phase-by-phase protocols, we've given you options from our line and, whenever possible, other brands that meet our standards as well.

If you hit your local health-food store on your own, these tips can help you select a good-quality supplement.

- **Look for the GMP** (good manufacturing practices) logo, and avoid supplements with dyes or artificial colors.

- **Find combination products.** Nutrients in a combination formula are often more effective or safer than one nutrient alone. For example, vitamin D products should contain vitamin K as well.

- **Natural doesn't always mean better.** "Food-based" supplements are intriguing and seem more "natural." They often contain common allergens such as soy, dairy, and gluten, and many times the synthetic form is better absorbed in your digestive track, so it's not a clear-cut advantage.

- **Choose a good green drink.** When choosing a powdered green drink, opt for a formula that is at least 50 percent organic and was processed with protection from UV light, heat, and moisture. (This ensures that the chlorophyll and nutrient content is maintained.) Avoid brands that have a lot of "fillers" such as lecithin, fibers, whole grasses, pectin, rice bran, or flax. Also avoid alfalfa-based formulas (if alfalfa is the first of several ingredients). Alfalfa can aggravate autoimmune conditions and is also a phytoestrogen, which can help or hinder your fat loss efforts, depending on your unique hormonal balance.

- **Buy only clean fish oil.** Ensure fish oil has been thoroughly tested for mercury and other heavy metals; is free of PCBs, pesticides, and dioxins; and is adequately preserved with antioxidants (you won't always be able to tell this from the label). The product should not smell overly fishy or be difficult to digest. Taking contaminated fish oil is worse than not taking any by a long shot. This is one area where store brands are not always a safe bet.

- **If taking vitamin E, select one with mixed tocopherols.** This means the supplement contains a blend of all four forms of naturally occuring vitamin E. Proportionately, the gamma tocopherol form should be largest, with low levels of the alpha form. The gamma form of vitamin E makes up 70 percent of our dietary intake of vitamin E, and supplements should mimic this ratio. Avoid vitamin E products that are "alpha-form" tocopherols only.

SMART WAYS TO STAY ON PLAN

Rank your adherence to the plan on a scale of 1 to 10. Every time you eat an item that's off plan (and we mean anything—a packet of regular sugar in your coffee, a tablespoon of ketchup on a burger, a piece of bread at a restaurant while you await your entrée), write it down in your Ultimate You Diet Diary (see page 259) and give each a value of 1.

At the end of each day, add the items up, subtract them from 10, and rank them as "X out of 10." For example, if you had half a sandwich and soup for lunch, that's 1 for the regular non-sprouted-grain bread, which is subtracted from 10 to give this day 9/10. Or if you had Cheddar cheese and bacon on your salad, you had 2 foods that are not on plan, making this day 8/10.

If you find that you are below 8 out of 10 at least 2 days per week, then you need to tighten the reins a bit to keep yourself losing. Review your food list and become

to keep it real, keep a food journal

You're busy. You're human. It's easy to forget that you grabbed a handful of M&M's as you passed a co-worker's desk, to recall sipping wine 2 nights last week when it was actually 4 nights, or to be unaware that you unconsciously reach for chocolate and caffeine every day at 3 p.m.

That's why on the Ultimate You plan you will keep a food journal. Yes, it may be tedious, but when you write down what you eat, you increase your awareness of what, how much, and why you are eating. In fact, one 2008 study, published in the *American*

Journal of Preventive Medicine, found that people who kept a food diary 6 days a week lost about twice as much weight as those who kept food records 1 day a week or less.

Use a journal of your own, or download the Ultimate You Diet Diary at www.bodybyhardware.com (see page 259 for a sample).

Keep a journal for several weeks, and see what you glean from it. If you are struggling with this process, visit us at www.bodybyhardware.com for customized coaching.

more familiar with the foods that we recommend you avoid. This system doesn't count your cheat meal. Remember, you should be on plan 90 percent of the time for fat loss, 75 to 80 percent for maintenance.

To troubleshoot challenges that can derail your ability to stay on plan, answer the following questions each time you choose an off-plan food.

- Did you eat it to indulge a craving?

- Did you eat it because you were hungry? Ravenous?

- Did you eat it because you were low in energy?

If you answered yes to any of the above, check your Diet Diary and examine your previous meal.

- Did it contain protein? Fibrous veggies? If not, add them into your next meal and ask the same questions. If yes, increase both at your next meal.

- Did it include a high-fiber, Optimal carb? If not, add 4 to 6 bites of a high-fiber carb to your next meal and reassess.

- Are you drinking enough water? Typically, 3 to 4 liters is enough for most women.

To know if a meal agreed with you, answer the questions below when you're finished eating.

- How is your sense of well-being? Is it low or "off"?

- Do you feel sleepy? (This is a key symptom in insulin resistance; see page 54 for more information.)

- Do you have any digestive upset—bloating, excessive fullness, diarrhea?

If you answered yes to any of the above:

- Eat more slowly, and consider a digestive enzyme formula such as Ultimate Digestizymes (Hardware).

- Ensure that your carbs were from the Optimal list for high-fiber starches.

- Use your Ultimate You Diet Diary to track which proteins best agree with you. You may find that you feel best on grass-fed beef rather than chicken or that you do well on fatty fish like salmon.

To keep it real, keep a food journal.

GET READY FOR BIG CHANGES

You will be doing this program on your own, so use these tools to track your progress.

Purchase a scale that tests body fat. While not perfectly accurate, measuring body fat has some advantages over merely watching the scale. The Tanita Ironman BC-549 is a good, all-inclusive model. Relying on the number on a regular scale will be frustrating, as there will be times you do not lose a pound, but swap a pound of fat for a pound of muscle. You will also occasionally gain water weight after a long flight, with PMS, or from lack of sleep, alcohol, more dairy or wheat, or too many carbs. Knowing these new pounds are water and not fat is very reassuring and can help you adjust your plan to get back on track. We recommend you weigh yourself and check body fat once per week, first thing in the morning and always on the same day, such as Monday morning. For body-fat scales, hydration matters, so follow water intake guidelines that come with your scale.

Take waist and hip measurements. They can show progress when the scale isn't moving—that's often much-needed motivation! We recommend the Gullick II tape measure (www.fitnessmart.com) to take accurate measurements. At the very least, take these measurements before you begin the program and then at the end of each phase. The key to accuracy is to take them at the exact same spot each time—you'll get the hang of it!

Follow these guidelines.

- **Waist:** Measure around the smallest part of your torso, usually about halfway between the bottom of your sternum/breastbone and your belly button.
- **Abdomen:** Place the tape at your belly button.
- **Hips:** Use the widest part of your hips, usually around the bony protuberance at the outside of your hip.
- **Thigh:** With legs slightly apart, measure at the widest part of your thigh, below the gluteal fold.
- **Calf:** Measure around the widest span.
- **Upper chest:** Measure at the fold where your chest and armpit meet.
- **Lower chest:** Measure at nipple level.

Judge other "nonscale" gains. Don't underestimate changes beyond pounds and percentages. Take note of all the gains you are making.

- Are you sleeping better?

- Is your skin clearer and brighter?

- Is your PMS improved or nonexistent?

- Do you recover faster from your workouts?

- Do you look less puffy?

- Do you feel more flexible and stronger?

- Are you more comfortable exercising or more at home in the weight room?

- Did you push through on a day when it felt really tough?

- Did you have a workout where you had perfect form on a tough exercise?

- Are you feeling stronger and more confident doing difficult exercises like squats?

- Do your dynamic warmups feel like less work?

WHEN THE GOING GETS ROUGH

Being your very best will be amazing—but it won't always be easy. There will be days when the thought of eating another chicken breast makes your stomach turn and the idea of sprinting on the treadmill makes you want to cry. At those times when a cupcake is calling your name, take these steps to pull through.

Are you having a tough day? Slow down and take a deep breath. Then take another. The cupcakes aren't going to help you . . . not really. Remind yourself of your Ultimate You. You want to fit into those jeans and lower your blood pressure, remember?

Are you hungry? If you haven't eaten in over 4 hours, you may be hungry. Also, if your last meal or your day in general lacked protein, fiber, and good fats or if you ate carbs that were not on plan, you may be battling a craving. Try these solutions to bust a craving.

- 16 ounces water—hunger is often dehydration in disguise; always start here, especially if you're low in water intake that day

- 1 to 2 teaspoons natural, unsweetened nut butter—lick it off a spoon like an ice cream cone, so you eat it slowly enough to have the fat signal hunger hormones to help you feel satisfied

order out the ultimate you way

If you dine out (or take out) more than you cook, you'll need to change how you order. Have a selection of menus that support your nutrition plan. You won't have control over the quality of protein you get or the kind of fat used in cooking, but this is the real world.

If you really want to stick to the program to the letter, here's some food for thought: Many restaurants now have more organic and free-range options, so seek them out. Also remember some dining-out basics: Choose grilled or baked versus fried; ask for double veggies instead of starchy carbs like mashed potatoes; choose oil and vinegar to dress salads instead of premixed salad dressings, or order those dressings on the side; avoid the bread basket before the meal; skip cream-based sauces and soups; add a small green salad to any entrée; and don't be afraid to ask the chef to prepare something to meet your needs.

If you're headed out on the town, the following cuisines fare well for your plan.

- **Greek:** Opt for grilled fish and shellfish entrées with a tomato and cucumber salad over doughy dishes like moussaka and spinach pie.

- **Italian:** Choose fish and chicken dishes and fresh basil and tomato salads while passing on pasta and breads.

- **Continental American:** Choices include salads, steaks, burgers (no bun), and many varieties of grilled chicken dishes. Skip the french fries and starchy side dishes like pasta or potato salads.

- **Thai:** This can be tricky—many Thai curry sauces have a fair amount of sugar, so skip those (or make your own at home with xylitol), and select any number of stir-fried options that include veggies and protein. Serve over a bed of baby spinach or steamed veggies and skip the rice. Pass on noodle dishes and fried rice.

- **Middle Eastern:** You have tons of great options: grilled kebabs with salads, fresh tomatoes, cucumbers, and low-fat feta cheese. Skip couscous, pita, and other bready items like kibbe and falafel.

- **Mexican:** Go grilled: Have the grilled fajitas without the tortilla, or experiment with other shrimp and fish options. Skip the rice and refried beans (refried beans are typically made with lard)—opt for black beans as a high-fiber carb, if they are available. Watch the cheese and sour cream here—they really add up! Go for guacamole instead.

- **Chinese:** Typically, Chinese restaurant sauces are loaded with sugar, cornstarch, and various other no-no's—not to mention sodium. Try no-sauce vegetable and protein options, steamed or stir-fried.

- ½ cup heavy cream with or without xylitol and cinnamon and 5 to 10 grams L-glutamine (do not use if you're insulin resistant or sensitive to dairy)

- 1 tablespoon vegetable-and-fruit-based fiber powder mixed in at least 8 ounces water

- ½ avocado (plain or try with balsamic vinegar and sea salt)

- 5 to 8 olives

- A protein snack, such as 3 ounces turkey or 2 hard-boiled eggs

Are you stressed? If so, your body will crave fatty and starchy foods—often in combination, such as baked goods or potato chips. Raising blood sugar and insulin is your body's way of lowering stress hormones like cortisol. (Remember, cortisol's job is to raise blood sugar, which can't stay low during a stressful situation. Traditionally, the response was to fight or flee a stressor, so your chemistry turns on the cravings for high-calorie foods to get fuel back up.)

Also, when you are under stress, you are burning up the feel-good brain chemical known as serotonin. Ever notice that when you eat a big plate of pasta, you feel very sleepy and relaxed afterward? That's the serotonin effect. One of the most efficient ways your body has to raise serotonin is to eat a meal high in carbohydrates—hence the craving for sugary or starchy foods and the calm, happy, sometimes sleepy, relaxed feeling after eating.

WHEN A CRAVING GETS THE BEST OF YOU

It finally happened: You slipped and ate the chips. You caved and ate the cupcake. What now?

Maybe you're the type who lets one slipup throw you completely off course. That's very common—we see it every day with our clients. They have one bagel when they're exhausted or one brownie when they feel blue, and a complex set of emotions comes into play.

Self-correction is the key to long-term success.

I blew it! they tell themselves, followed by *Well, today's ruined; I'll start again tomorrow.* If the slip happens on a Friday, it's *I've totally messed up; I'll get back on track on Monday.* Sound familiar?

See what happened? That one bagel or brownie went from one unhallowed carb to a whole day or even an entire weekend of being off plan. Bagels, cupcakes, and potato chips will happen—just don't let them derail you for days on end. Self-correction is the key to long-term success.

Another common self-defeating behavior: You let one slip turn on the "beat yourself up" talk in your head. Giving in to a craving can easily start a downward spiral of negative self-talk and guilt that gets you "all down in it," as we call it. When you are down in it, you wallow in the guilt over bad food choices or beat yourself up for missing a workout. Then you're unable to make good food choices at your next meal because you feel terrible about yourself and your fat [insert body part of choice here].

> When you start the negative talk, spin it positively by repeating your mantra to yourself 10 times.

Don't let guilt set in. Learn to control the negative chatter in your head. It is tough and it takes practice, but it can be done. Try this: Have a clear, present-tense, positively stated mantra that affirms your Ultimate You, such as "I am so happy and comfortable in my lean, healthy body." When you start the negative talk, spin it positively by repeating your mantra to yourself 10 times. If you don't feel better, repeat it another 10. If the idea of your Ultimate You is still foreign to you, it may be helpful to do this practice 1 to 3 times daily until you believe it.

Some days you just need a cookie. If you decide to have one, own that choice. Decide you are going off plan, make a conscious decision to indulge, and make a conscious decision to get back on track. So long as you are consciously making the decision, you are in control.

After your cookie, forget it and get back on track. Make your next meal a good one and get to the gym. Your Ultimate You is waiting.

CHAPTER 8

Phase 1: Preparation

WHETHER YOU'RE AN EXERCISE NEWBIE or have been training for a while, Phase 1 will teach you to work out using correct technique and to rest and recover from that work. You'll also introduce basic lifestyle changes and learn to train with your mind, as well as with your muscles.

That's it, but that's plenty.

Depending on your current fitness level, Phase 1 can be either a challenge or a breeze. (Please note: If you have any ankle, knee, hip, back, or shoulder injuries, please consult your doctor or an appropriate health professional before you perform any of these exercises.) If it's too easy, use heavier weights and/or step up the intensity of the cardio, but don't skip this phase. Even if it doesn't seem very difficult, it's still new to your muscles on a neurological level. We're talking about working *movements,* as well as working muscles.

> Train with your mind, as well as with your muscles.

Here's the core concept: Eat better, move smarter. You have to learn to do both of these things, and you must progress in stages. You crawl before you walk, walk before you jog, jog before you run, run before you sprint, right? Phase 1 gives you the fundamental exercises, tools, and techniques you'll need to continually take your body and workout to the next level—not just now but for life.

Rest assured: Though basic, Phase 1 training will change your body. But as you burn calories, burn fat, and lose inches, you'll move better and increase the ability of your body to do more work, whether that's doing household chores with increased energy and endurance or improving your fitness level for your weekend tennis game.

ULTIMATE YOU WORKOUT
Get Acclimated to Training

In Phase 1, your goals are to increase your base conditioning, core strength, and muscular endurance. To meet these goals, you'll train five times a week—three strength-training sessions and two EST sessions. You can train at the gym or at home, and we've structured the workouts so that they're adaptable to your schedule and life . . . so no excuses!

To refresh your memory, the Ultimate You workout contains three elements. Here's a recap.

- STRENGTH-TRAINING: While the strength-training exercises are important, so are the movements that precede them. Always perform the dynamic warmup, which primes your joints and muscles for work, and the activation drills, which "wake up" muscles that are typically underutilized and/or inherently weak.

- EST: The object is to build an aerobic base so you can transition into more-demanding EST sessions, which will ultimately help you get leaner. The EST sessions in Phases 2 through 4 will put higher demands on your muscular and cardiovascular systems, which will force your body to expend more calories and take longer for them to return to *homeostasis* (resting state).

- RECOVERY: Always foam roll after each workout in both your EST and resistance-training sessions. Perform static stretching after each EST session, and feel free to do it after resistance-training sessions, too (after you've foam rolled). You can also perform foam rolling before the dynamic warmup of the resistance-training session, particularly if you're feeling sore or tight. And feel free to incorporate some other recovery techniques from Chapter 4 as well. Remember: Muscles repair, rebuild, and strengthen when you rest, not when you train.

ULTIMATE YOU NUTRITION
Clean Up Your Diet

- Master two key meals: breakfast and your splurge meal.

- Dial in meal timing, and get enough sleep to improve levels of growth hormone and leptin.

Set Up for Success

- Establish a regular meal schedule. Eat every 3 to 4 hours, and make sure each meal contains protein, veggies/fiber, and carbs from the Optimal or Allowable lists.

- Glance at the recipes in the Appendix. Use them to create quick meals and menus that keep your taste buds happy.

- Troubleshoot common problems. If you can't eat in the morning or you overeat in the evening, skip meals, or eat out often, brainstorm solutions or try ours.

- Start your basic supplement regimen. It will help reduce food cravings, enhance your body's ability to burn fat, and boost your energy and overall health.

PHASE 1 WORKOUT AT A GLANCE

During Phase 1, you'll alternate between the strength-training workout (Strength 1) and the EST workouts that you'll find on page 122, taking 2 days for recovery and regeneration.

- HOW LONG: 4 weeks
- HOW OFTEN: 5 workouts a week
  - 3 Phase 1 strength-training sessions (Strength 1)
  - 2 EST sessions (see page 122)
- GOALS: To increase base conditioning, core strength, and muscular endurance

WEEK	MONDAY	TUESDAY	WEDNESDAY	THURSDAY	FRIDAY	SATURDAY	SUNDAY
1	Strength 1	EST-1	Strength 1	EST-1	Strength 1	Off	Off
2	Strength 1	EST-2	Strength 1	EST-2	Strength 1	Off	Off
3	Strength 1	EST-3	Strength 1	EST-3	Strength 1	Off	Off
4	Strength 1	EST-4	Strength 1	EST-4	Strength 1	Off	Off

PHASE 1 STRENGTH-TRAINING PROGRAM

Dynamic Warmup

	Sets	Reps	Load	Tempo	Rest	Intensity
A: Side Lying 90-90 Stretch	1	5/side	b/w	Slow	10 sec	Low
B: Forward Lunge	1	5/side	b/w	Slow	10 sec	Low
C: Lateral Squat	1	5/side	b/w	Slow	10 sec	Low

Activation Drills

	Sets	Reps	Load	Tempo	Rest	Intensity
A: Standing Single-Leg External Rotation with Mini-Band	1	6/side	TBD	2-0-1-1	10 sec	Low
B: Floor W	1	6	b/w	1-0-1-1	10 sec	Low

Strength Training

	Sets	Reps	Load	Tempo	Rest
A1: Swiss Ball/Body-Weight Squat	2–3	↑15	TBD	3-1-1-0	60 sec
A2: Pushup	2–3	↑15	b/w	2-0-1-0	60 sec
B1: Supine Glute Bridge with Mini-Band	2–3	↑15	TBD	2-0-1-1	60 sec
B2: Reverse-Grip Lat Pulldown	2–3	12–15	TBD	3-0-1-1	60 sec
C1: Prone Pillar Bridge—modified	2–3	TBD	b/w	↑30 sec hold	60 sec
C2: Prone Back Extension	2–3	TBD	b/w	↑30 sec hold	60 sec

strength-training dictionary

Set: The number of times a particular exercise will be performed.

Repetition ("rep"): The number of times a movement will be performed within a set.

Repetition maximum (RM): The number of reps per set that can be performed at a given resistance with proper technique.

Load: The amount of weight or resistance being used. Load is determined by the number of reps in the range. Exercises that require you to choose a weight will be noted under the column load with *TBD* (to be determined). Picking resistance is not an easy task and is dictated by the repetition bracket. If the repetition bracket is 10 to 12 RM (repetition maximum), then the resistance chosen should allow you to perform 10 repetitions with perfect form at a minimum and 12 repetitions with perfect form at a maximum. If you can't perform 10 reps, the resistance is too heavy; if you can perform 13 reps, the resistance is too light.

Rest period (or recovery): The time—in seconds, minutes, hours, or days—between repetitions, sets, training sessions, etc. Recovery can be static (complete rest) or dynamic (active recovery).

Tempo: The speed of movement. Tempo is defined by four numbers separated by dashes. This technique was pioneered by world-renowned strength-training coach Charles Poliquin. More information is available at www.charlespoliquin.com.

- The first number represents the *eccentric movement* (the lowering of the weight).
- The second number represents the length of the pause in the muscle's lengthened position.
- The third number is the *concentric movement* (the raising of the weight).
- The last number is the length of the pause the muscle is in the contracted position before the movement is repeated.

To perform an exercise with a 3-1-1-0 tempo:

1. **Lower** the weight for 3 seconds. (3)
2. **Pause** in the lengthened position for 1 second. (1)
3. **Raise** the weight for 1 second. (1)
4. **Do not pause** in the contracted position. (0)

Sequence: This refers to the order of exercises. Exercises that are listed by letter/number combination (A1/A2, B1/B2, etc.) comprise a sequence. They are meant to be performed in succession. For example, here's a sample sequence from the strength-training section of the chart to your left: Complete up to 15 reps (1 set) Swiss Ball/Body-Weight Squat (A1) and rest 45 to 60 seconds; next, complete up to 15 reps (1 set) Pushup (A2), and rest 45 to 60 seconds. Repeat this process another 2 or 3 times (as indicated in the Sets column) before moving on to the next sequence of exercises (B1/B2 and C1/C2).

PHASE 1 STRENGTH TRAINING
Dynamic Warmup

A: Side Lying 90-90 Stretch

LOCATION: HOME OR GYM

This exercise opens up the chest muscles and warms up the muscles that rotate the torso for movement, such as the obliques.

Sets: 1
Reps: 5 per side
Load: Body weight
Tempo: Slow
Rest interval: 10 seconds
Intensity: Low

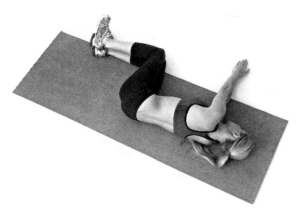

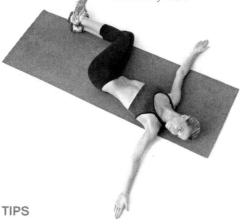

START POSITION

LIE on your right side.

STACK your legs so that they form 90° angles at the knee and hip joints.

STACK your shoulders so that your upper arms form a 90° angle with your torso, and place your palms on top each other.

THE MOVEMENT

LIFT your left arm and reach back; try to touch the floor on your left. Rotate your torso only.

RETURN your left arm to the start position. With each repetition, try to open up your chest and spinal muscles a little more.

PERFORM 5 repetitions on your right side, then repeat on your left side.

TIPS

PLACE a rolled-up towel under your neck for extra support. Advanced: To strengthen your neck muscles, raise your head slightly off the floor.

AS you rotate, let your head follow your arm.

TRY placing a rolled-up towel or piece of foam between your knees and press against it as you work.

KEEP your knees on the ground throughout the exercise.

YOU may notice that one side of your torso feels tighter than the other. If so, add 1 or 2 extra reps on the tighter side.

B: Forward Lunge

LOCATION: HOME OR GYM

This movement lengthens the anterior hip and thigh muscles of the trailing leg and strengthens the quadriceps, hamstrings, and glutes of the front leg.

Sets: 1
Reps: 5 per side
Load: Body weight
Tempo: Slow
Rest interval: 10 seconds
Intensity: Low

START POSITION

STAND with your feet about hip-width apart, chest up, shoulders back, abdomen pulled in, head and spine in good alignment.

PLACE your hands on your hips for balance.

THE MOVEMENT

WITH your left foot, step forward about 2 to 3 feet. Plant your left foot flat; make sure your weight is on the heel of that front foot. Raise the heel of your right foot so that you're balancing on your toes.

BEND your rear knee and front leg and slowly lower your torso straight down to the floor until your rear knee is 2 inches from the floor. The knee of the trailing leg should be at a 90° angle with the floor and your front thigh at a 90° angle with your torso.

Note: If your flexibility allows, you can extend your trailing leg further behind you to deepen the stretched position.

STEP back and return to the start position. Perform 5 repetitions on your left side, then repeat with your right leg.

TIPS

MAKE sure your weight is on the heel of your front foot. You should be able to wiggle your toes in the bottom position.

TRY to drop down without moving your knee past the middle of your foot.

TO improve balance, you may perform this exercise with one hand against a wall or hold a dowel rod like a staff.

C: Lateral Squat

LOCATION: HOME OR GYM

This movement lengthens the inner thigh muscles (adductors) of the trailing leg and strengthens the glutes, quadriceps, and hamstrings of the front leg.

Sets: 1
Reps: 5 per side
Load: Body weight
Tempo: Slow
Rest interval: 10 seconds
Intensity: Low

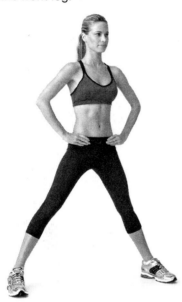
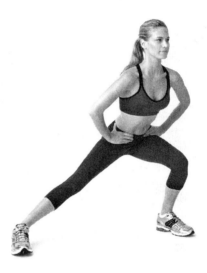

START POSITION

STAND with your feet about hip-width apart, hands at your sides.

LIFT your head and chest, draw your shoulders down and back, and place your spine in good alignment.

PLACE your hands on your hips and step to the right about 2 feet.

THE MOVEMENT

BEND your knee and start to lower your hips by sitting back rather than down (i.e., bend your knee and start to push your hips backward). Keep your chest high and your spine in proper alignment, but angle your torso forward slightly.

AT the bottom of the movement, pause. You should feel a stretch in the inner thigh of your opposite leg.

RETURN to the start position.

PERFORM 5 repetitions with that leg, then repeat with your other leg.

TIPS

FOR better balance, perform this exercise with your arms and hands extended in front of you, or you can hold a dowel rod like a staff for balance.

AS you bend your knee, keep it squarely over your toes—don't let it cave in or bow out.

BEGIN this exercise with your less-dominant leg first (for most people, the less-dominant leg is the one they wouldn't kick a ball with), and never train the stronger side more than the weaker side. If you can perform only 4 repetitions on your weak side, perform 4 repetitions on your strong side.

Activation Drills

A: Standing Single-Leg External Rotation with Mini-Band

LOCATION: HOME OR GYM

This drill strengthens the external rotators of the hip of the working leg.

Sets: 1
Reps: 6 per side
Load: To be determined
Tempo: 2-0-1-1
Rest interval: 10 seconds
Intensity: Low

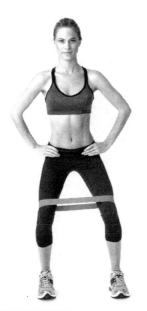 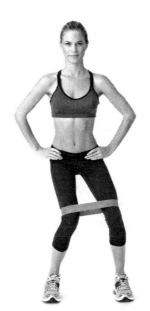 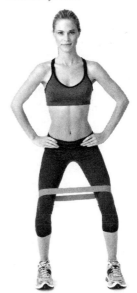

START POSITION

SLIP the band over both legs and position it slightly above your knees. Stand with your feet hip-width apart, chest up, shoulders back, and spine in proper alignment.

BEND your knees slightly and drop your hips back slightly, so your butt sticks out a bit.

PLACE your hands on your hips.

THE MOVEMENT

KEEPING both feet on the floor, dip your right leg and knee inward (from 2 to 5 inches, depending on your range of motion). Keep the tension in the band on the opposite side.

RETURN your right leg and knee to the start position, so you feel tension on the band on both sides. Perform 6 repetitions on your left side, then repeat with your right leg.

TIPS

START with your less-dominant leg.

ONE leg may feel stronger than the other. That's okay. The other side will get stronger over time.

B: Floor W

LOCATION: HOME OR GYM

This exercise activates the muscles of the upper back (rhomboids, trapezius, and posterior deltoids), as well as the external shoulder rotators.

Sets: 1

Reps: 6

Load: Body weight

Tempo: 1-0-1-1

Rest interval: 10 seconds

Intensity: Low

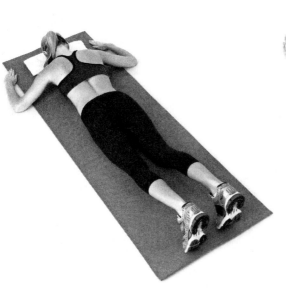 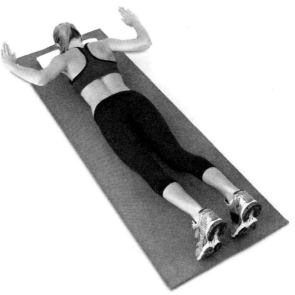

START POSITION

LIE facedown with your arms outstretched so that your forearms are parallel to each other and your palms flat on the floor. (From above, your upper arms, forearms, and hands should form a W.)

FLEX your feet to engage your shin muscles.

THE MOVEMENT

LIFT your chest and arms slightly—upper arms, forearms, and hands, still palms down—toward the ceiling. Keep your arms in the W position as you squeeze your shoulder blades down and back.

RETURN to the start position and repeat.

TIPS

PLACE a rolled-up towel under your forehead for comfort.

DON'T lift your head and chest too much. Let your arms perform most of the exercise.

REALLY squeeze your shoulder blades and lift those hands toward the ceiling—even slightly higher than the elbows, if possible.

Strength Training

A1: Beginner: Swiss Ball Squat

LOCATION: HOME OR GYM

This exercise targets the quads, hamstrings, and glutes.

   BEGINNERS: You may switch to the Body-Weight Squat at any time in weeks 2 to 4. Make sure you have the strength, flexibility, and stability to perform this exercise with good form.

Sets: 2 or 3
Reps: Up to 15
Load: To be determined
Tempo: 3-1-1-0
Rest interval: 60 seconds

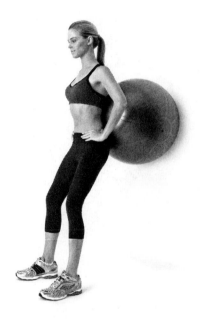

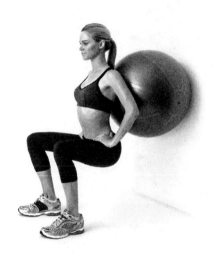

START POSITION

PLACE the ball against a wall, then place your back against the ball—position the apex of the ball at your lumbar spine. Walk your feet out about 18 inches.

CHECK your posture—lift your chest, draw back your shoulders, contract your abdomen.

THE MOVEMENT

BEND your knees and slowly lower your body to a count of 3. Your hips should be positioned slightly beneath the ball.

LET your body roll with the ball—when you reach 3, the apex of the ball should be behind your shoulder blades.

RETURN to the start position to a count of 1.

TIP

WHEN you can perform 3 sets of 15 reps with body weight, challenge yourself: Perform the exercise with 5-pound dumbbells. Hold a pair of dumbbells down by your thighs, palms in, chest up, arms straight, shoulders back.

A1: Intermediate/Advanced: Body-Weight Squat

LOCATION: HOME OR GYM

Sets: 2 or 3
Reps: Up to 15
Load: To be determined
Tempo: 3-1-1-0
Rest interval: 60 seconds

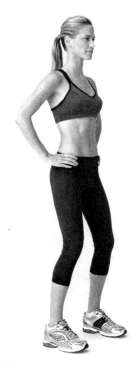

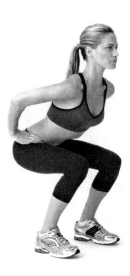

START POSITION

POSITION your feet slightly wider than hip-width apart; turn out your toes slightly.

THE MOVEMENT

SLOWLY bend your knees, pushing your hips back as you do so. Continue to lower your body as far as you can without lifting your heels off the floor. Pause.

PUSH your weight back up to return to the starting position.

TIPS

KEEP your chest up, shoulder blades retracted, and maintain a neutral lumbar spine.

IMAGINE that you are lowering yourself onto a small stool.

IF you can't perform the movement without your heels coming off the floor, try putting a couple of 5- or 10-pound plates under your heels. Stretch your calves and hamstrings. If they are tight, that might be the reason your heels are coming up.

WHEN you can perform 3 sets of 15 reps with body weight, challenge yourself: Perform the exercise with 5-pound dumbbells. Hold a pair of dumbbells down by your thighs, palms in, chest up, arms straight, shoulders back.

A2: Pushup

LOCATION: HOME OR GYM

This exercise targets the upper body (pecs, anterior deltoids, and triceps) and the muscles of the core.

Three choices for three levels of fitness:

Sets: 2 or 3
Reps: Up to 15
Load: Body weight
Tempo: 2-0-1-0
Rest interval: 60 seconds

1. If you don't yet have the upper-body strength for a regular pushup, try a modified pushup on your knees.
2. The Power-Rack Pushup (in the gym; see page 116) offers a great way to progress toward performing a regular pushup.
3. If you are at an intermediate/advanced level of fitness, start with regular pushups.

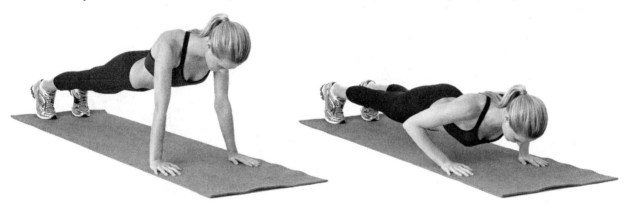

START POSITION

PLACE your palms flat on the mat, your hands slightly wider than shoulder-width apart, and your fingers facing forward or slightly inward.

SLOWLY shift your weight forward until your shoulders are positioned directly over your hands. Fully extend your body without any bend at the hips or knees.

CONTRACT your abdominals, glutes, and quadriceps and align your head with your spine.

MODIFIED pushup: Begin as above but with your knees and feet on the floor.

THE MOVEMENT

SLOWLY lower your body toward the floor, keeping your torso still. Try to form a 45° angle between your upper arms and your torso.

CONTINUE to lower yourself until your chest or chin touches the mat. Allow your elbows to flare outward as you lower.

PRESS straight up to return to the start position.

TIPS

LOOK down as you lower and lift.

TRY to move your torso and hips as a chain—don't let your body sag.

PUSH through the heel and outside surface of your palm—this gives more force in your press and greater stability to your shoulders.

WHETHER you perform the regular or modified pushup, as soon as you can no longer keep your spine and core in alignment, stop the set.

A2: Power-Rack Pushup

LOCATION: GYM

Sets: 2 or 3
Reps: Up to 15
Load: To be determined
Tempo: 2-0-1-0
Rest interval: 60 seconds

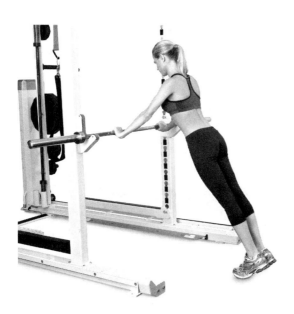
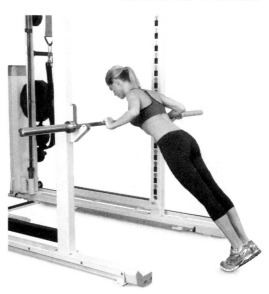

START POSITION

PLACE your hands slightly wider than shoulder-width apart on a power rack. Keep your feet together and point your toes toward your shins. Position your shoulders directly over your hands.

FULLY extend your body as in a standard pushup. Your shoulders, spine, hips, knees, and ankles should be in a straight line that angles downward from shoulders to ankles.

CONTRACT your abdominals, glutes, and quadriceps and align your head and spine.

THE MOVEMENT

SLOWLY lower your body toward the bar, keeping your torso still and in good alignment.

CONTINUE to lower yourself until your chin is aligned with the bar. Allow your elbows to flare outward as you lower.

PRESS straight up to return to the start position.

TIPS

LOOK down as you lower and lift, not up or straight ahead.

TRY to move your torso and hips as a unit. Think of your body as a chain—don't let it sag.

B1: Supine Glute Bridge with Mini-Band

LOCATION: HOME OR GYM

This exercise targets the hamstrings, glutes, and lower back.

Sets: 2 or 3

Reps: Up to 15

Load: To be determined

Tempo: 2-0-1-1 (intermediate/ advanced: for each rep, you can work up to a 3- to 5-second hold at the top of the movement)

Rest interval: 60 seconds

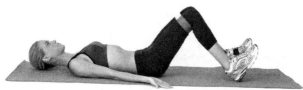 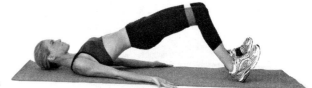

START POSITION

POSITION your mini-band just above your knees. Lie on your back, arms at your side, palms facing the ceiling.

BEND your hips and knees, feet flat on the floor, heels 6 inches from your butt.

MOVE your feet about 12 inches apart so that you cause tension in the band. Bring your toes toward your shins so you're on your heels only.

THE MOVEMENT

MAINTAINING proper form and a straight spine, press your heels into the floor as you lift your hips off the floor.

COME all the way up so your knees, hips, and shoulders form a straight line. Keep your

abdomen nice and tight and continue to pull your toes toward your shins.

PAUSE and then lower back to the floor.

TIPS

KEEP your toes pulled toward your shins throughout the exercise.

MAKE sure you press down through your heels while trying to extend your knees away from your hips.

AT the top of the movement, your knees, hips, and shoulders should form a straight line.

MAKE sure you press your legs slightly out against the mini-band throughout the movement.

B2: Reverse-Grip Lat Pulldown

LOCATION: GYM

This exercise targets the lats and biceps.

Sets: 2 or 3

Reps: 12 to 15

Load: To be determined

Tempo: 3-0-1-1

Rest interval: 60 seconds

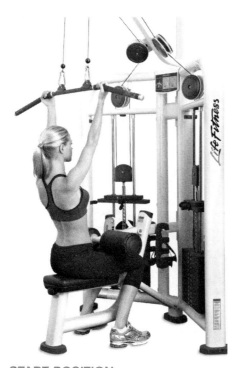
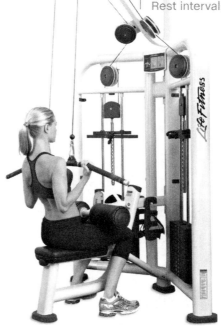

START POSITION

ADJUST the plates to the desired weight. Sit tall facing the machine. Adjust the thigh pads.

STAND and grasp the bar with your hands shoulder-width apart and palms facing you.

PULL down the bar and sit, thighs under the pads, knees bent 90 degrees, feet flat on the floor.

LEAN slightly backward and extend your arms, but keep your elbows soft.

THE MOVEMENT

PULL the bar down until it touches your upper chest. Imagine that invisible hands are under your elbows and you're pressing down and in

against them. Press down and in throughout the downward phase. Pause.

RETURN to the start position. Repeat to complete the set.

TIPS

THROUGHOUT the exercise, keep your wrists straight.

AS you lower the bar, keep your spine straight. Do not swing or lean back.

IF you start to round the upper back, you're using too much weight.

AS you perform the exercise, imagine someone has their hands under your elbows. Press against those invisible hands.

B2: Reverse-Grip Lat Pulldown with Tubing

LOCATION: HOME

Sets: 2 or 3
Reps: 12 to 15
Load: To be determined
Tempo: 3-0-1-1
Rest interval: 60 seconds

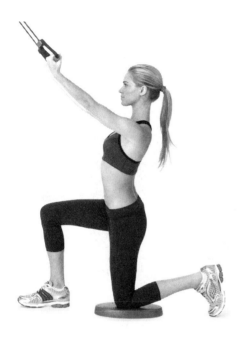
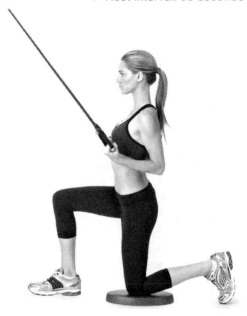

START POSITION

LOOP one end of the tubing around a stationary object or doorjamb. Tug a few times to ensure that the tubing is securely fastened.

GET on one knee. Your forward knee makes a 90° angle with the floor. Kneel on your rear knee with your toes on the floor. (Place a towel under your rear knee for comfort.) Lift your chest and keep your spine straight.

GRASP the end of the band with your palms and arms facing the ceiling.

LEAN back slightly and extend your arms in front of you, above shoulder height and possibly above your head, depending on how high you've secured the tubing.

THE MOVEMENT

BEND your elbows and slowly pull them back alongside your body, so that your elbows end up behind your torso. Keep your wrists locked so that your forearm and the back of your hand form a straight line.

RETURN to the start position. Repeat to complete the set.

TIPS

AS you pull, lead with your elbows. Imagine trying to get your elbows to touch behind your back.

AS you pull, keep your torso still. Only your arms should move.

C1: Prone Pillar Bridge

LOCATION: HOME OR GYM

Beginner: Modified plank position (on knees)

Intermediate/advanced: Full plank position

This exercise targets the abdominals, primarily as stabilizers.

Sets: 2 or 3

Reps: To be determined; work up to 30-second hold

Load: Body weight

Rest interval: 60 seconds

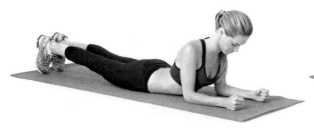 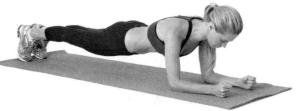

START POSITION

LIE facedown, legs straight out behind you, knees and feet together. Bend your elbows, with your forearms facing each other, and support your weight on your forearms. Form loose fists.

LIFT yourself to your knees, toes on the floor.

CONTRACT your abdominal muscles and arch your torso up off the mat.

THE MOVEMENT

KEEP your abdominal muscles tight and raise your knees off the floor to a pushup position, forming a straight line from your head to your heels. (If you are a beginner, you may keep your knees on the ground.) Hold.

RETURN to the start position.

TIPS

CORRECT form is important. It's better to perform more reps with shorter holds than to do one 30-second rep with bad form. If possible, perform this exercise in front of a mirror to ensure proper form.

OVER the course of Phase 1, work up to 1 repetition, held for 30 seconds.

KEEP your elbows under your shoulders throughout the exercise.

C2: Prone Back Extension

LOCATION: HOME OR GYM

This exercise improves posture, strengthens the muscles of the lower and upper back, and helps prevent future back pain.

Sets: 2 or 3

Reps: To be determined; work up to 30-second hold

Load: Body weight

Rest interval: 60 seconds

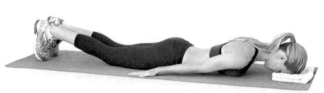 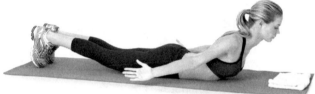

START POSITION

LIE on your stomach with your arms to the sides, hands flat on the floor, toes on the floor.

THE MOVEMENT

STARTING with your head and upper back, raise your torso off the floor until your chest comes off the ground while rotating your arms so that your palms are facing away from your body. Hold for up to 30 seconds using good form.

RETURN slowly to the start position.

TIPS

KEEP your head, neck, and spine in a straight line throughout the exercise.

KEEP your shoulders down and your neck long.

Energy System Training: Treadmill*

LOCATION: HOME OR GYM

*If you don't have access to a treadmill at home, walk outdoors. Refer to the RPE and HR training zone charts on pages 28 and 29.

Note: Increase treadmill speed up to 4 mph for all workouts.

WEEK 1 (ALL LEVELS, 21 MINUTES TOTAL), EST-1

WARMUP: 3 minutes, 3 to 3½ mph, 0 incline

WORKOUT: 15 minutes (zone 2, RPE 3 to 4, 0 incline)

COOLDOWN: 3 minutes, 3 to 3½ mph, 0 incline

WEEK 2
BEGINNER: 26 MINUTES TOTAL, EST-2

WARMUP: 3 minutes, 3 to 3½ mph, 0 incline

WORKOUT: 20 minutes (zone 2, RPE 3 to 4, 0 incline)

COOLDOWN: 3 minutes, 3 to 3½ mph, 0 incline

INTERMEDIATE/ADVANCED: 21 MINUTES TOTAL, EST-2

WARMUP: 3 minutes, 3 to 3½ mph, 0 incline

WORKOUT: 180 seconds of work; increase the incline of the treadmill so that heart rate rises to zones 2 to 3 (RPE 3 to 6), followed by 120 seconds of recovery; decrease incline of treadmill to 0 so that heart rate falls back to zone 1 (RPE 1 to 2); repeat 3 times.

COOLDOWN: 3 minutes, 3 to 3½ mph, 0 incline

WEEK 3
BEGINNER: 24 MINUTES TOTAL, EST-3

WARMUP: 3 minutes, 3 to 3½ mph, 0 incline

WORKOUT: 180 seconds of work; increase incline of treadmill so that heart rate rises to zones 2 to 3 (RPE 3 to 6), followed by 180 seconds of recovery; decrease incline to 0 so that heart rate falls to zone 1 (RPE 1 to 2); repeat 3 times

COOLDOWN: 3 minutes, 3 to 3½ mph, 0 incline

INTERMEDIATE/ADVANCED: 22 TO 26 MINUTES TOTAL, EST-3

WARMUP: 3 minutes, 3 to 3½ mph, 0 incline

WORKOUT: 180 seconds of work (increase incline of treadmill so that heart rate rises to zones 2 to 3, RPE 3 to 6), followed by 60 seconds of recovery (decrease incline of treadmill to 0 so that heart rate falls to zone 1, RPE 1 to 2); repeat 4 or 5 times

COOLDOWN: 3 minutes, 3 to 3½ mph, 0 incline

WEEK 4
BEGINNER: 26 MINUTES TOTAL, EST-4

WARMUP: 3 minutes, 3 to 3½ mph, 0 incline

WORKOUT: 120 seconds of work (increase incline of treadmill so that heart rate rises to zones 2 to 3, RPE 3 to 6), followed by 120 seconds of recovery (decrease incline of treadmill to 0 so that heart rate falls to zone 1, RPE 1 to 2); repeat 5 times

COOLDOWN: 3 minutes, 3 to 3½ mph, 0 incline

INTERMEDIATE/ADVANCED: 24 TO 27 MINUTES TOTAL, EST-4

WARMUP: 3 minutes, 3 to 3½ mph, 0 incline

WORKOUT: 120 seconds of work (increase incline of treadmill so that heart rate rises to zones 2 to 3, RPE 3 to 6), followed by 60 seconds of recovery (decrease incline of treadmill to 0 so that heart rate falls to zone 1, RPE 1 to 2); repeat 6 or 7 times

COOLDOWN: 3 minutes, 3 to 3½ mph, 0 incline

ENERGY SYSTEM TRAINING POST-WORKOUT

FOAM rolling sequence (pages 42 to 45)

STATIC stretching (pages 45 to 47)

the mind/body connection in action

Years ago, before I got really into training, I read about how using your mind as you train—you might call it mindfulness—can maximize your results. But when I heard trainers say things like "Oh, the mind is very powerful," I kind of laughed.

My problem with this idea was that many of the people who espoused it were so out there in their presentation that it seemed comical rather than valid science. But once I really got into training, I stopped laughing.

There's tons of research that shows that thinking about your movements when you train can stimulate the nervous system even more.

When I train, I focus on several things.

- **Posture:** I'm always thinking about maintaining good posture when I train.

- **Movement:** I focus on good form, on executing each movement in the proper way.

- **Resistance:** I make sure the load I'm using directly opposes that movement pattern.

- **Core engagement:** I think about engaging my core, and matching that engagement to the weight and resistance I'm using. For example, if I'm using 45-pound dumbbells, I don't need to tighten my core like I'm lifting a 300-pound barbell.

Your "core" is all the muscles from your hips to your ribs, stretching all the way around from front to back (basically, belly button to backbone). Engaging your core means keeping that area in a neutral position (not bent forward, back, or side to side) and tight (think of tightening or bracing to take a punch to the gut). If you glance in a mirror, you might even notice your belly sticks out a bit when you engage it, rather than sinking in.

Focus on *tempo*. When you are mindful of tempo, you focus on each rep. You may start out really thinking about tempo: "Lower the weight for 3 seconds, pause for 1 second, and then raise for 1 second." But eventually you'll streamline it to "3, 2, 1, hold, 1, up, 1." That's your mind ruling your body and your body responding to your mind.

That's the mind/body connection in action. Remember to work your body as rigorously as you work your mind and eventually you'll reap the benefits.

As you become more familiar with the movements of each exercise and with training in general, they will become second nature.

—Joe Dowdell

PHASE 1 NUTRITION
Phase 1 at a Glance

WEEK 1

- Learn to put a meal together.
- Eat breakfast.
- Enjoy your splurge meal!

WEEK 2

- Add basic supplements to your program.
- Plan ahead.

WEEK 3

- Fine-tune your meal timing.
- Get good-quality sleep.

WEEK 4

- Transition to Optimal foods.

In Phase 1, you'll begin to balance hormones that play a critical role in regulating appetite and body composition. These hormones—leptin, glucagon, and growth hormone—work when your blood sugar is lower and when you sleep. Fortunately, they all respond well to lifestyle changes and diet.

If you currently eat many of the foods on the Ultimate You food list, choose more Optimal, rather than Allowable, foods. If you don't, simply eat the foods on the plan, and don't worry whether they're Optimal or Allowable. You'll make that shift in Phase 2.

Also, don't panic if you don't lose a significant amount of weight or body fat in the next 4 weeks. Follow Phase 1 to the letter and you're likely to lose more fat, more easily, in Phases 2 through 4.

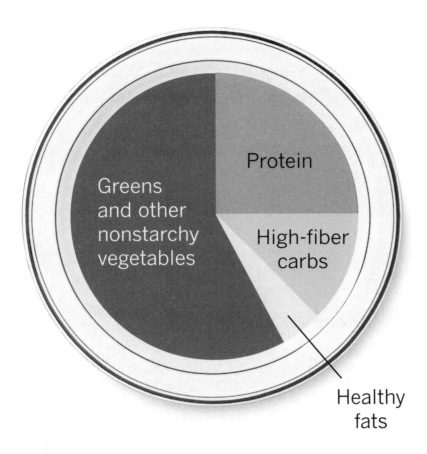

Week 1

LEARN TO PUT A MEAL TOGETHER

If proteins are the bricks of your meal, vegetables are the mortar. A higher-protein diet needs lots of green and brightly colored veggies to alkalinize and provide fiber (refer to the plate graphic above). The easiest way to put your meal together is to put protein over a bed of vegetables. Alternatively, just over half of your plate should be covered in vegetables (e.g., a chicken breast beside a large salad).

You will always have a full 4- to 6-ounce serving of lean protein. Include some healthy fats (such as olive oil on the veggies, a small handful of nuts, or half an avocado). When you include a high-fiber carbohydrate, follow these guidelines.

- 4 bites (or ⅓ cup) to 6 bites (½ cup) of legumes, pumpkin, sweet potato, etc.

- 4 to 6 bites or up to 1 slice of sprouted-grain or hemp bread

- 2 high-fiber crackers (e.g., GG Crispbread, FiberRich, Wasa, or Ryvita)

- ½ cup of berries or 1 medium apple or pear

perk up your morning appetite

Did you eat dinner too late? Have a cocktail or two later in the evening? Did you sleep poorly, or are you stressed out? Any one of these issues can dampen hunger in the morning.

Your liver "cleans house" when you sleep. If it must work on dinner or detox alcohol, it can't do its other jobs, and you awaken less than eager to eat again.

Also, when you have food in your system at bedtime, leptin and growth hormone can't rise. When this happens, it is harder to regulate your appetite the next day and harder to lose body fat.

If you're not hungry in the morning, try these tips.

- Have a glass of lemon water as soon as you get up. This stimulates digestion.

- Start your breakfast with a piece of high-fiber fruit.

- Try the whey protein shake in the Appendix (page 278).

- Before bed, down this concoction: Mix 1 scoop of Ultimate Cleanse liver-cleanse beverage and 1 tablespoon of non-grain-based fiber powder (see recommended brands on page 66) in 1 cup of water or coconut water. Take it until your morning appetite picks up, or—because it provides excellent liver support—make it part of your bedtime routine.

- If none of the above options perk up your desire for breakfast, particularly for a protein-based breakfast, you may have abnormal morning cortisol levels. Consider discussing this with a nutritional medicine practitioner, but know you'll learn a lot about managing cortisol in Phase 2.

See the Appendix on page 275 for meal ideas and recipes, as well an overview of a typical day on the plan.

EAT BREAKFAST

Eat breakfast within an hour of getting out of bed, unless you exercise first thing in the morning. You *must* consume protein at every meal, including breakfast. The Ultimate You breakfast includes lean protein and veggies. Eggs are the most palatable protein choice for most people, but feel free to eat any lean Optimal or Allowable protein.

You may have noticed that, other than whole or steel-cut oats, there are no cereals on this plan. Despite marketing claims, cereals do not have nearly enough fiber and nutritional value to offset their carbohydrate content. While they are quick, if you get up just 15 minutes earlier, you'll have time to cook and enjoy a great breakfast, and you'll be set up to burn fat for the rest of the day.

Don't have time to make breakfast, you say? You can whip up any one of the tasty meals in the Appendix (see page 275) in 10 minutes. And while it might seem strange to eat a small green salad in the morning, you might soon crave it. But to get used to breakfast veggies, start adding bell peppers, onions, mushrooms, prewashed baby spinach, and so on to omelets and scrambles.

ENJOY YOUR SPLURGE MEAL!

On the Ultimate You plan, you can look forward to one splurge meal each week. Not only is this meal a mental break from the parameters of the plan, but this larger meal (higher in calories and carbs) also resets leptin, which reins in cravings and hunger for the upcoming week. It also helps spur the thyroid to keep metabolism revved high—so don't skip it! Use this meal to eat something that you are missing on the plan. Go ahead and order the pasta if you've been feeling deprived. Or have dessert. But be careful not to overdo it by gobbling up fried calamari followed by lasagna and a piece of cake. Use this meal to break from the plan—but if you go too hog wild, you'll miss the mark.

FYI: You may feel excessively full or simply not so good right after a splurge meal or the next morning, especially if your indulgence contained lots of starchy carbs, was heavy in fat, or included alcohol. While this reaction isn't unusual, you'll likely be reminded that when you eat well, you feel great.

Week 2
ADD BASIC SUPPLEMENTS TO YOUR PROGRAM

The Ultimate You plan suggests specific supplements for each phase. These supplements target and help rebalance specific hormones, including estrogen, cortisol, and others.

The brands below meet high standards of efficacy and safety.

- Hardware: available at www.bodybyhardware.com

- Designs for Health: available at www.designsforhealth.com and www.bodybyhardware.com

- Poliquin Performance: available at www.charlespoliquin.com

To give you more options, additional brands and over-the-counter products are suggested whenever appropriate as well.

The Phase 1 supplement prescription includes three basics.

1. A high-quality multivitamin/mineral formula. So you won't lose water-soluble vitamins in your urine—or have trouble digesting a jam-packed tablet—opt for a multivitamin capsule formulated to be taken two or three times a day with food, rather than a "one-a-day."

A word about iron: Most menstruating women can safely take a multi that includes this mineral. But to be certain, do not supplement with iron unless you've assessed your iron needs via a blood test and it's been recommended to do so by your health-care provider.

Products: Formulated to curb cravings and manage insulin, Ultimate Metabolic Multi (Hardware) is an ideal multi that supports weight loss (take 2 capsules at each meal, 6 per day). Other quality multivitamin brands, available at most health-food stores, include Jarrow, Nature's Way, and Blue Bonnet.

2. A high-quality fish-oil supplement. Choose one that contains high levels of EPA/ DHA. Start with 1 gram of EPA/DHA with food 3 times a day, and work up to 2 grams with meals 3 times per day (thus, 6 grams daily).

If you "retaste" or burp after you take your fish-oil supplement, it's probably of poor quality. If this happens and you take a brand suggested here, you might have trouble digesting fat and might benefit from a digestive-enzymes formula such as Ultimate Digestzymes or a liver-gallbladder formula such as LVGB Complex (Designs for Health).

Products: Try Ultimate Omega 3 (Hardware) or Ultimate Omega (Nordic Naturals).

3. Antioxidant support with a powdered greens drink. Stress, environmental pollution, your immune system, and even your workouts generate free radicals that can cause damage in your body. You have elaborate internal systems of antioxidant support, and it's wise to support those systems to stay energetic, healthy, and young.

An easy, effective way to get a full range of antioxidants is to use a high-quality greens product such as Ultimate Greens (Hardware) or Primal Greens (Poliquin Performance). Take at least 1 tablespoon twice daily mixed in water. (It's safe to take up to 5 tablespoons per day.)

If you prefer a capsule, choose a brand that contains a variety of antioxidants such as grapeseed extract, resveratrol, ginkgo biloba, curcumin, quercetin, lycopene, EGCG (from green tea), vitamin C, vitamin A, alpha-lipoic acid, CoQ10, and vitamin E (in the form of mixed tocopherols).

Products: Look for Ultimate Anitox (Hardware), Resveratrol Synergy (Designs for Health), or Grapeseed Supreme (Designs for Health). Take 1 to 3 capsules daily or as directed on the bottle.

PLAN AHEAD

You schedule in time for important appointments and workouts, right? It makes sense to make time to plan and prepare your meals, too. Spend an hour on a Saturday afternoon or Sunday evening prepping food for the week ahead, and you'll save time and increase your odds of success.

There's more you can do than precut veggies, too.

- Steam or quickly stir-fry hearty veggies like kale, Swiss chard, asparagus, broccoli, asparagus, cauliflower, and carrots. These will keep in the fridge for at least a week.

- Stir-fry sliced chicken breasts (or bake whole ones) for easy salads during the week.

- Broil several lean beef or bison patties to top a salad, make a quick snack, or have as your breakfast protein.

- Hard-boil 6 to 12 eggs to add to salads or for easy protein snacks. Or make a large Veggie Frittata or Spinach Timbales (recipes on pages 276 and 287) and store in the fridge for quick protein-veggie meals or snacks that are great cold or warmed up.

- Bake several sweet potatoes. Wash, poke holes in them with a fork, wrap in foil, and bake at 400°F for about 45 minutes (until you can easily poke through the skin with the fork).

Even if you cook every night for your family, you can still prep your own meals. Here's how you might utilize these prepped foods.

- **Breakfast:** Quickly sauté a handful each of prechopped mushrooms and pre-washed spinach, then add eggs or egg whites for a scramble—prep and cook time under 5 minutes.

> Stay on a regular meal schedule because it is crucial for success.

- **Lunch:** Throw 3 large handfuls of prewashed lettuce and a handful of chopped bell peppers into a glass Pyrex dish. Drizzle with olive oil and balsamic vinegar, throw in sliced prebaked chicken breast, and voilà! You've prepped a lovely salad for lunch in about 2 minutes.

- **Snack:** Steam 10 asparagus spears and hard-boil 2 eggs, and you've got a veggie-protein snack ready in under a minute.

- **Dinner:** Throw a handful of prechopped veggies such as onion, bell peppers, celery, and zucchini into a frying pan with 1 tablespoon of coconut oil, then quickly stir-fry until the veggies just change colors; serve alongside a precooked bison burger, and there's dinner in about 5 minutes.

Week 3
FINE-TUNE YOUR MEAL TIMING

It can be a challenge, but get on—and stay on—a regular meal schedule because it is crucial for success. With several days of perfectly timed meals under your belt, you'll feel satisfied and in control of your hunger.

worried by a 3-hour meal window?

If you've followed the "eat every 2 hours" advice and worry that you can't go longer than that—or if you find yourself hungry, light-headed, dizzy, or sleepy soon after you eat—ask yourself the following: At your last meal, did you:

■ . . . eat enough protein?

■ . . . eat any foods that you know you are sensitive to or allergic to, such as wheat, dairy, soy, or another known allergen?

■ . . . eat plenty of vegetables and fiber?

■ . . . eat not-so-healthy carbs? That is, were they low-fiber, simple carbs like bread, bagels, pasta, pastries, or sugar?

Also ask yourself:

■ Do I get enough sleep?

■ Do I drink more than 1 to 2 cups of coffee per day?

■ Are my adrenals weak or tired? Only a qualified health professional can tell you for sure, but if you're under chronic stress or have had trouble keeping your blood sugar up in the past, this may be the case.

■ Am I insulin resistant? (See Chapter 5.)

Address these issues, and you won't sacrifice one hormone imbalance for another.

How often to eat? You may have heard or read that it's desirable to eat every 2 hours. But eating too frequently, and thus releasing insulin every 2 hours all day, can cause insulin resistance and an exaggerated insulin response that thwarts your body's ability to burn fat and enhances its ability to store it.

What's more, when blood sugar is elevated, glucagon and growth hormone will not rise. That's not good—just as we need fuel several times per day, we need times of low fuel as well. The trick is not to let the interval between meals get too long, which can cause an exaggerated cortisol (stress) response.

On this program, you'll eat every 3 to 4 hours. This allows your body to better absorb, digest, and utilize your last meal and allow your blood sugar to lower, but not by too much. It also helps your body build or maintain lean muscle mass as it breaks down fat. If you listen to your body and stay on plan, you're likely to feel hungry in about 3 hours anyway.

> Eat every 3 to 4 hours: breakfast, midmorning snack, lunch, midafternoon snack, and dinner.

Typically, though, eating too often isn't the problem—it's getting caught up in a busy day, so you either don't make time or forget to eat. If this sounds like you, schedule your mealtimes into your day—literally. You might use the scheduling software on your computer or set the alarm on your cell phone.

what's the skinny on alcohol?

Here's what happens to your metabolism when you drink.

- **You stop burning fat at the cellular level.** The body can't store alcohol. So when it's ingested, it's metabolized before anything else. Every other calorie—from fat, sugar, whatever—gets put on hold. You are now set up to store fat, rather than burn it.

- **Your blood sugar lowers abruptly.** Alcohol temporarily "paralyzes" your liver's ability to make its own sugar (*gluconeogenesis*), which indirectly causes a drop in blood sugar. When this happens—and especially if you drink on an empty stomach—you end up ravenous. Further, because of its effect on blood sugar, alcohol may cause you to wake in the night, or first thing in the morning, ravenous and with a craving for simple carbs like cereal, pancakes, or waffles.

- **Your growth hormone drops.** Alcohol causes this directly, and because its metabolites are stimulants, and it wreaks havoc on your blood sugar, it can also affect sleep. Lack of sleep also affects growth hormone as well as leptin, which leaves you hungrier the next day.

- **Your testosterone plummets.** Alcohol increases the conversion of testosterone to estrogen in body fat, a process called *aromatization*. If you are overweight and/or you have any issues with your menstrual cycle or low sex drive—just to name a few problems—then you are at least relatively estrogen-dominant, and alcohol will be an even bigger issue for you.

The bottom line: Limit alcohol to one or two times a week, opt for red wine or "clear drinks" like vodka soda with lime or olives, and avoid sugary cocktails like margaritas. Also, drink an additional liter of water to counteract dehydration, eat lean protein and veggies with your hooch, and skip carbs at meals that include alcohol.

You've heard about the benefits of drinking red wine in moderation. The problem with drinking in moderation: Some people can't do it. If you're one of them, skip booze for now and tackle moderate drinking during your maintenance phase.

SIMPLE MEAL-TIMING TIPS

- Eat every 3 to 4 hours: breakfast, midmorning snack, lunch, midafternoon snack, and dinner.

- On strength-training days, your post-workout Recovery Shake counts as one of your snacks.

- Eat your last meal 2 to 3 hours before bedtime or at least 12 hours before breakfast. This is important because your liver needs to do its detox work, not digest dinner, and your blood sugar levels need to come down to stimulate normal leptin and growth hormone secretion. Your body also needs to fast at night to have a normal appetite and appropriate cortisol response in the morning.

If you have a social event that will keep you eating past 8 p.m., these tips can help.

- *Option 1:* Eat a larger second lunch or early dinner rather than an afternoon snack. If dinner is served, choose light veggie-protein appetizers rather than a large entrée.

- *Option 2:* Have a larger "second lunch" in the late afternoon, and skip food entirely at the event. When you get home, have "dinner" as a protein shake to which you've added 1 tablespoon of non-grain-based powdered fiber. (You digest liquid meals more quickly.)

   If you must eat a larger meal, skip alcohol or stick to one glass of wine. Alcohol will slow your digestion of dinner (because it has to be metabolized first), and you'll be headed to bed with a full belly, which hinders leptin and growth hormone.

GET GOOD-QUALITY SLEEP

You know how important sleep is to recovery and regeneration, but lack of sleep can trigger hunger and cravings as well. Poor sleep is often tied to an abnormal stress response, in which the natural rhythm of cortisol is disrupted or there is an abnormal secretion of adrenaline, both due to tired adrenal glands (see Phase 2). Stress also depletes serotonin, a calming brain chemical. If you have trouble falling asleep, try these tips at night to bolster the production of serotonin in the evening.

- One hour before bed, stop working—that means put away the office paper-work, bills, or vacuum cleaner. If you want to read to relax, choose something light (and definitely not work-related or a suspenseful page-turner).

> Make most, if not all, of your high-fiber carb choices non-grain-based.

- Dim your lights. Low-light lamps or candles are ideal.

- If you watch TV to relax, turn the rest of the lights off.

- Be sure your bedroom is quiet, not too hot or too cold, and block out as much light as possible.

- If you tend to wake up hungry at night, take 1 tablespoon of non-grain-based fiber mixed in water at bedtime. Or 30 minutes before you turn in, have ½ scoop of whey powder mixed with water or coconut water.

If these natural remedies don't work, consult a nutritional medicine practitioner who can help restore your natural hormonal rhythms, or speak with your doctor about a sleeping medication. It's more detrimental to not sleep than to take a sleep aid. (And fear not—you'll tackle cortisol in Phase 2.)

dine out without freaking out

Until this becomes a way of life, it may be easier to eat more meals at home, where there is less temptation. However, nearly all of our clients live in New York City, and many of them eat very few, if any, meals prepared at home—and they are still successful with this plan. Here are a few tips to keep in mind.

- Start each meal with a big glass of water and a side salad.

- Order a salad and a protein appetizer instead of a larger entrée.

- Choose proteins and vegetable-based options, or ask for double veggies instead of the starch. And ask the waiter not to bring the bread basket.

- Get sauces on the side.

- Look for broiled, baked, poached, or grilled options over fried ones.

- Don't be afraid to ask if an entrée can be prepared differently to suit your needs.

- Since most restaurants don't offer grass-fed beef and bison, opt for fish—a nice piece of grilled fish is one of the leanest proteins you can eat.

Week 4

TRANSITION TO OPTIMAL FOODS

You've now had nearly a month on a high-plant, high-protein diet with only high-fiber carbs. You're eating better than you have in years. Now you'll make a few shifts to help your body burn fat even better. From now on:

1. Make most, if not all, of your high-fiber carb choices non-grain-based and from the Optimal list. These include sweet potatoes, yams, pumpkin, winter squashes, and legumes. Also, limit or avoid sprouted-grain products and high-fiber crackers, and fine-tune your portions—4 to 6 bites (⅓ to ½ cup) of high-fiber starch is ideal.

2. Consider dairy a condiment rather than a protein choice. It's fine to have 1 to 2 tablespoons of low-fat cheese on eggs or a salad a couple of times per week, but don't rely on yogurt or cottage cheese for a protein serving.

> Choose the leanest, highest-quality cuts of protein available.

3. Choose the leanest, highest-quality cuts of protein available, and watch consumption of fattier, saltier meats, such as turkey bacon, chicken or turkey sausage, deli meats, and conventionally raised animals. Try to limit these to once per week, if you have them at all.

4. Limit nuts to ¼ cup and nut butters to 1 tablespoon per serving. Also, try spreading nut butter on a celery stick or an apple, rather than on a slice of hemp bread or Wasa cracker.

5. Eat more green vegetables. Yes, *more*. Continually look for opportunities to add more veggies to both breakfast and snack choices. (For example, you might add a side salad to every lunch or dinner that is not a salad.) If you can't stomach more green veggies, have a serving of your green drink 1 or 2 times a day.

CHAPTER 9

Phase 2: Accumulation

IN PHASE 2, YOU'LL WORK out more days and increase the intensity of both your strength training and EST. Your goals are to increase lean muscle mass, decrease body fat, and utilize anaerobic interval training. You'll train 6 times a week—3 strength-training sessions, 2 EST sessions, and 1 EST recovery session. As in Phase 1, you can train at the gym or at home.

ULTIMATE YOU WORKOUT

Here's your Phase 2 workout in a nutshell. Don't worry—you're ready!

- **STRENGTH TRAINING:** You will alternate between two different strength-training programs: A and B. Each week, one of the programs will get a higher priority, and you will perform it twice that week. As in Phase 1, always perform the dynamic warmup and activation drills. While the dynamic warmup remains the same for both Programs A and B, the activation drills will change between each program so that you can target different areas.

- **EST:** In the EST portion of this phase, you'll begin anaerobic intervals. As we mentioned earlier, the literal meaning of *anaerobic* is "without oxygen." Anaerobic exercise means you're working at such a high level of intensity that your cardiovascular system can't deliver oxygen to your muscles fast enough. Because your muscles need oxygen to continue to work, anaerobic exercises only last for short bursts.

However, the benefits are enormous. This type of training raises your metabolic rate from a steady fire to a blazing burn. Anaerobic intervals allow your body to achieve maximum caloric expenditure throughout the workout. They also increase your body's metabolic disturbance, so you'll burn more calories post-workout for up to 48 hours. When you do anaerobic intervals, you definitely want to stay in your target heart-rate zone.

You'll do from 19½ to 27 minutes, including warmup and cooldown, on a stationary bike, using your unique heart-rate and RPE training zones. These workouts will intensify each week, which will ultimately help you get leaner.

You'll also perform a weekly EST recovery workout for 36 to 55 minutes (including warmup and cooldown) of a low-intensity steady-state cardio session, such as a brisk walk or slow jog.

- RECOVERY: Always foam roll after each workout in both your EST and resistance-training sessions. Perform static stretching after each EST session, and feel free to do it after resistance-training sessions, too (after you've foam rolled). You can also perform foam rolling before the dynamic warmup of the resistance-training session, particularly if you're feeling sore or tight. And feel free to incorporate some other recovery techniques from Chapter 4 as well. Remember: Muscles repair, rebuild, and strengthen when you rest, not when you train.

ULTIMATE YOU NUTRITION
Rev Up the Fat-Burning Process

In Phase 2, you will begin to tighten up your diet and increase your body's sensitivity to insulin. You'll do this by selecting more foods from the Optimal list, reducing your intake of dairy products, and managing your carbohydrates at each meal. For the insulin-resistant, you'll avoid raising insulin at the start of your day by focusing on lean protein and healthy fats at breakfast. With insulin under control, you'll burn more fat all day.

Tweak Hormones to Your Advantage

You'll learn to prevent insulin from rising too much after meals, while taking advantage of its ability to support recovery and lower cortisol after your workouts. We'll show you how to raise your cortisol level when you train (one of the few times high cortisol is desirable), then bring it down afterward—and how to keep it in check the rest of the day.

Chill Out and Choco Up

In Phase 2, you'll learn to manage stress to shed fat more easily—and indulge in our delicious Ultimate You cocoa recipes. What's not to love?

PHASE 2 WORKOUT AT A GLANCE

We've designed 2 separate strength-training routines for this phase: Programs A and B. For the next 4 weeks, you will alternate between them.

The EST workouts will be different with the exception of the recovery session, which will remain the same for the rest of the process.

- HOW LONG: 4 weeks
- HOW OFTEN: 6 times a week
  - 3 Phase 2 strength-training sessions
  - 2 EST sessions
  - 1 EST recovery session
- **Goals:** To increase lean muscle mass; decrease body fat; introduce anaerobic interval training

WEEK	MONDAY	TUESDAY	WEDNESDAY	THURSDAY	FRIDAY	SATURDAY	SUNDAY
1	Strength 2-A	EST-5	Strength 2-B	EST-5	Strength 2-A	EST-R	Off
2	Strength 2-B	EST-6	Strength 2-A	EST-6	Strength 2-B	EST-R	Off
3	Strength 2-A	EST-7	Strength 2-B	EST-7	Strength 2-A	EST-R	Off
4	Strength 2-B	EST-8	Strength 2-A	EST-8	Strength 2-B	EST-R	Off

PHASE 2 STRENGTH-TRAINING: PROGRAM A

Dynamic Warmup

	Sets	Reps	Load	Tempo	Rest	Intensity
A: Side Lying 90-90 Stretch	1	5/side	b/w	Slow	—	Low
B: Forward Lunge with Elbow to Instep	1	5/side	b/w	Slow	—	Low
C: Handwalk—Forward	1	4–5	b/w	Slow	30 sec	Low

Activation Drills

	Sets	Reps	Load	Tempo	Rest	Intensity
A: Glute Bridge— Mini-Band	1	10–12	TBD	2-0-1-1	—	Low
B: Floor T	1	6	b/w	1-0-1-1	—	Low

Strength Training

	Sets	Reps	Load	Tempo	Rest
A1: Split Squat	3	10–12/side	TBD	3-0-1-0	45 sec
A2: Flat Dumbbell Bench Press	3	10–12	TBD	3-0-1-0	45 sec
B1: Supine Swiss Ball Leg Curl	3	10–12	b/w	2-0-2-0	45 sec
B2: Seated Row for Upper Back	3	10–12	TBD	2-0-1-1	45 sec
C1: Side Pillar Bridge— Kneeling	3	10–12/side	b/w	2-0-1-1	45 sec
C2: 45° Back Extension	3	10–12	b/w	2-0-1-1	45 sec

PHASE 2 STRENGTH TRAINING: PROGRAM A
Dynamic Warmup

A: Side Lying 90-90 Stretch

LOCATION: HOME OR GYM

This exercise opens up the chest muscles and warms up the muscles that rotate the torso for movement, such as the obliques.

Sets: 1
Reps: 5 per side
Load: Body weight
Tempo: Slow
Rest interval: —
Intensity: Low

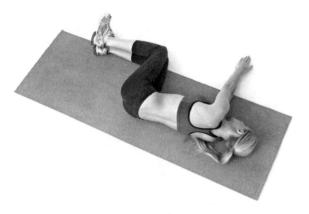
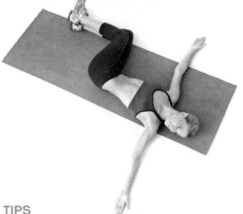

START POSITION

LIE on your right side.

STACK your legs so that they form 90° angles at the knee and hip joints.

STACK your shoulders so that your upper arms form a 90° angle with your torso, and place your palms on top each other.

THE MOVEMENT

LIFT your left arm and reach back; try to touch the floor on your left. Rotate your torso only.

RETURN your left arm to the start position. With each repetition, try to open up your chest and spinal muscles a little more.

PERFORM 5 repetitions on your right side, then repeat on your left side.

TIPS

PLACE a rolled-up towel under your neck for extra support. Advanced: To strengthen your neck muscles, raise your head slightly off the floor.

AS you rotate, let your head follow your arm.

TRY placing a rolled-up towel or piece of foam between your knees and press against it as you work.

KEEP your knees on the ground throughout the exercise.

YOU may notice that one side of your torso feels tighter than the other. If so, add 1 or 2 extra reps on the tighter side.

B: Forward Lunge with Elbow to Instep

LOCATION: HOME OR GYM

This exercise stretches the groin, hip flexors, and quadriceps of the trailing leg and strengthens the glutes, quadriceps, and hamstrings of the lead leg.

Sets: 1	
Reps: 5 per side	
Load: Body weight	
Tempo: Slow	
Rest interval: —	
Intensity: Low	

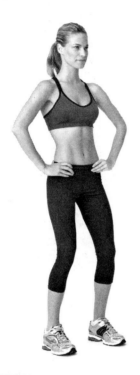

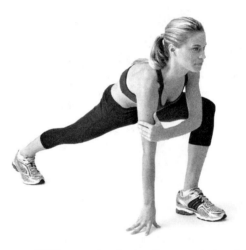

START POSITION

STAND with your feet together.

THE MOVEMENT

WITH your left foot leading, step into a lunge, keeping your trailing leg as straight as possible.

PLACE your left elbow to the inside of your left shin. Then place your left hand on your right elbow. Place the fingers of your right hand on the ground, in line with your left foot.

LIFT your chest, stand up, and step into the next repetition with your right leg.

REPEAT to complete the set.

TIPS

KEEP your back knee off the ground.

SQUEEZE your back glute during the stretch.

KEEP your torso and chest upright as much as you can.

C: Handwalk—Forward

LOCATION: HOME OR GYM

This exercise elongates your hamstrings, calves, and lower back and engages the shoulders and core as stabilizers.

Sets: 1

Reps: 4 or 5

Load: Body weight

Tempo: Slow

Rest interval: 30 seconds

Intensity: Low

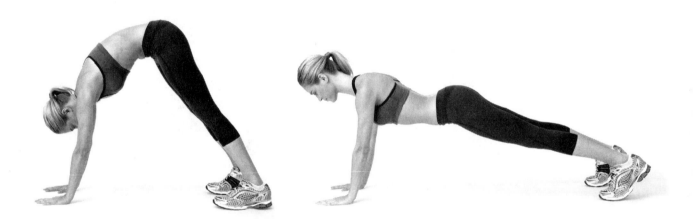

START POSITION

STAND tall with your legs straight and your stomach tight.

BEND forward at the waist and place your hands on the floor.

THE MOVEMENT

WALK your hands away from your legs, keeping your stomach tight, and try to keep your heels on the ground as long as you can. You should feel a pleasant stretch in your calves, hamstrings, and lower back.

SLOWLY walk your hands forward until you reach your limit, without allowing your midsection to dip toward the floor. Then walk your feet back in toward your hands.

MAKE sure you take very small steps (i.e., inch forward).

TIP

IF you aren't yet flexible enough to touch your toes, find your start position by walking your hands out in front of you as far as you can while still keeping your heels on the floor.

Activation Drills

A: Glute Bridge—Mini-Band

LOCATION: HOME OR GYM

Sets: 1
Reps: 10 to 12
Load: To be determined
Tempo: 2-0-1-1
Rest interval: —
Intensity: Low

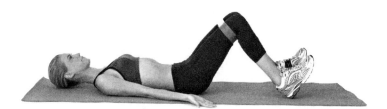

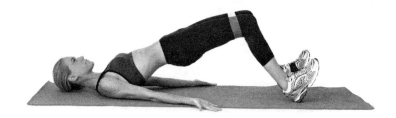

START POSITION

POSITION your mini-band just above your knees. Lie on your back, arms at your side, palms facing the ceiling.

BEND your hips and knees, feet flat on the floor, heels 6 inches from your butt.

MOVE your feet about 12 inches apart so that you cause tension in the band. Bring your toes toward your shins so you're on your heels only.

THE MOVEMENT

MAINTAINING a straight spine, press your heels into the floor as you lift your hips off the floor.

COME all the way up so your knees, hips, and shoulders form a straight line. Keep your abdomen nice and tight.

PAUSE, then lower back to the floor.

TIPS

PRESS down through your heels while trying to extend your knees away from your hips.

AT the top of the movement, your knees, hips, and shoulders should form a straight line.

B: Floor T

LOCATION: HOME OR GYM

This exercise activates the back of the shoulders (posterior deltoids) and the upper back (rhomboids and trapezius muscles) and elongates the pecs and front of the shoulders (anterior deltoids).

Sets: 1

Reps: 6

Load: Body weight

Tempo: 1-0-1-1

Rest interval: —

Intensity: Low

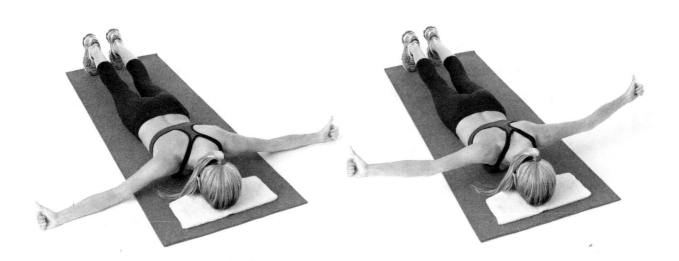

STARTING POSITION

LIE facedown on the floor.

THE MOVEMENT

DRAWING your shoulder blades in toward your spine, extend your arms to the sides to create a T shape with your arms and torso. Keep your thumbs up.

KEEP your arms straight and your thumbs toward the ceiling.

RETURN to start position. Repeat to complete the set.

TIPS

KEEP your abdominals tight and your thumbs raised throughout the exercise.

KEEP your neck long and your shoulders down.

Strength Training

A1: Split Squat

LOCATION: HOME OR GYM

This exercise targets the quadriceps, hamstrings, glutes, and adductors of the lead leg.

Sets: 3
Reps: 10 to 12 per side
Load: To be determined
Tempo: 3-0-1-0
Rest interval: 45 seconds

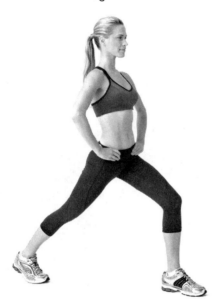 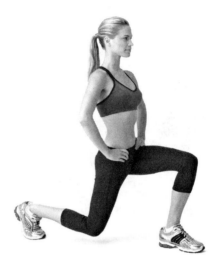

START POSITION

STAND with your hands on your hips or hold dumbbells (if you're using them) at your sides.

KEEPING your torso vertical, position your forward leg so that your weight falls through the heel of your front foot. Raise your back foot, so your heel is off the floor and some of your weight is supported on the ball of your foot.

THE MOVEMENT

SLOWLY bend your rear knee; shift your front knee forward, and lower your torso straight to the ground so that your rear knee is about 2 inches from the floor. At the bottom position, make sure your front knee stays over the middle of your foot.

SHIFT your front knee forward, keeping it behind your toes.

REVERSE direction and return to the start position. Do the reps for the forward leg first, then switch legs and do the reps for your back leg.

TIPS

IF extra resistance is needed, hold dumbbells in each hand.

KEEP your chest up and your shoulders back.

ALIGN your head with your spine. Do not round or flex forward.

DON'T let your knee touch the floor.

A2: Flat Dumbbell Bench Press

LOCATION: HOME OR GYM
This exercise targets the pecs, anterior deltoids, and triceps.

Sets: 3	
Reps: 10 to 12	
Load: To be determined	
Tempo: 3-0-1-0	
Rest interval: 45 seconds	

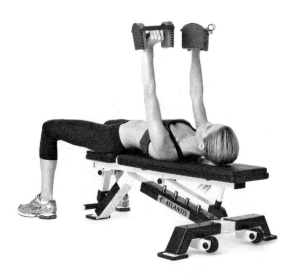 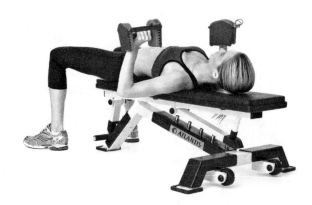

START POSITION
LIE on a flat bench, feet flat on the floor. Lift the weights up over your chest, your arms straight above your shoulders, with your knuckles facing the ceiling.

THE MOVEMENT
SLOWLY lower the dumbbells, keeping your arms at a 45° angle to your torso. Lower until arms are slightly lower than shoulder level, making sure to tuck your elbows.

PRESS dumbbells back up to the start position and repeat to complete the set.

TIPS
DRAW your shoulder blades together slightly.

DO not let your forearms pitch forward or backward—they should remain vertical.

TRY to keep the dumbbells aligned so that at the bottom of the movement, your hands are directly over your elbows.

B1: Supine Swiss Ball Leg Curl

LOCATION: HOME OR GYM

This exercise targets the glutes, hamstrings, lower back, and calves, as well as all the stabilizing musculature of the core.

Note: Perform this exercise on a nonslippery surface, such as a rubber mat.

Sets: 3
Reps: 10 to 12
Load: Body weight
Tempo: 2-0-2-0
Rest interval: 45 seconds

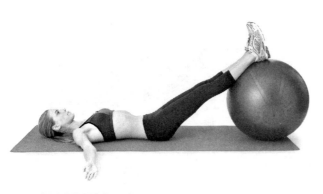
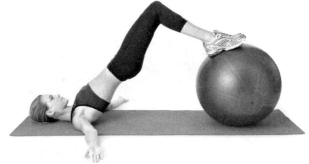

START POSITION

LIE on your back, your arms extended out to the side, palms facing up.

PLACE your heels on top of the ball, with your legs and feet together. Push your heels into the ball and your arms into the floor for stability.

THE MOVEMENT

CONTRACT your core and glutes, push your heels into the ball, and raise your hips off the floor as you continue to push down into the ball.

AT the top of the movement, your ankles, knees, hips, and shoulders should be in a straight line. Hold the position momentarily.

PULL your heels in toward your glutes as far as you can.

REVERSE the action. Think about extending your legs rather than pushing your feet.

BEGINNERS: Return to the initial start position.
INTERMEDIATE/ADVANCED: Keep your hips elevated for the duration of the set.

TIPS

THINK of this exercise as a series of commands: Raise up, pull in, squeeze, extend out, lower.

MAKE sure that the ball doesn't transition from one surface to another. For example, don't perform this exercise so that the ball moves from rubber mat to wood floor.

THE farther out your arms are to the side, the more balance you'll have. The closer in, the less balance you'll have, and the more challenging the exercise will be.

B2: Seated Row for Upper Back

LOCATION: GYM

This exercise targets the back of the shoulders (posterior deltoids) and upper back (rhomboids and trapezius).

Sets: 3	
Reps: 10 to 12	
Load: To be determined	
Tempo: 2-0-1-1	
Rest interval: 45 seconds	

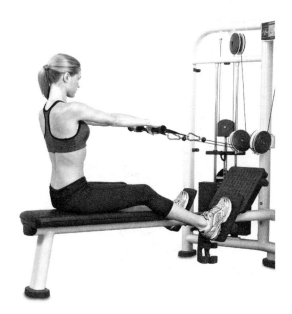 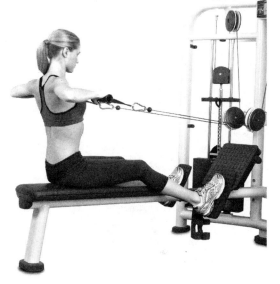

START POSITION

ADJUST the plates to the desired weight. Sit tall facing the machine—proper spinal alignment, chest lifted, shoulders down—and grasp the handles.

PLACE your feet on the platform high enough so that your weight pushes through your heels. Bend your knees slightly. Tighten your core muscles.

THE MOVEMENT

PULL back on the handles until your elbows are just past a 90° angle. Maintain proper spinal alignment and keep your torso vertical.

YOUR wrists should remain straight and your arms parallel to the floor throughout the entire movement.

RETURN to the start position. Repeat to complete the set.

TIPS

AS you perform the exercise, move your arms and shoulders only.

KEEP your shoulders down and fully retract your shoulder blades at the end of the movement.

B2: Seated Row with Resistance Tubing

LOCATION: HOME

This exercise targets the back of the shoulders (posterior deltoids) and upper back (rhomboids and trapezius).

Note: Different color tubing will correlate to more or less resistance.

Sets: 3	
Reps: 10 to 12	
Load: Body weight	
Tempo: 2-0-1-1	
Rest interval: 30 seconds	

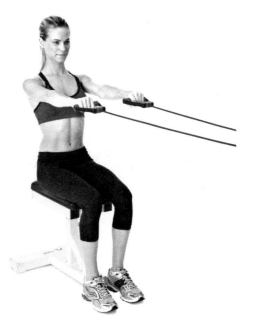 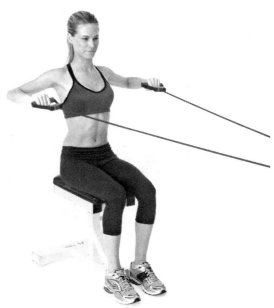

START POSITION

ATTACH the tubing to a secure object, such as a doorknob. Give a few tugs to make sure the tubing is securely fastened.

GRASP the handles, arms extended.

MAINTAIN proper spinal alignment, lift your chest, and draw your shoulders down and back.

PLACE your feet flat on the floor.

TIGHTEN your core muscles.

THE MOVEMENT

PULL back on the handles until your elbows are just past a 90° angle. Focus on maintaining good posture.

YOUR wrists should remain straight and your arms parallel to the floor throughout the entire movement.

RETURN to the starting position. Repeat to complete the set.

C1: Side Pillar Bridge—Kneeling

LOCATION: HOME OR GYM

This exercise—a modification of the side pillar bridge—targets the internal and external obliques, as well as the quadratus lumborum.

Sets: 3

Reps: 10 to 12 per side (intermediate/advanced: may hold for 3 to 5 seconds per rep)

Load: Body weight

Tempo: 2-0-1-1

Rest interval: 45 seconds after completing both sides

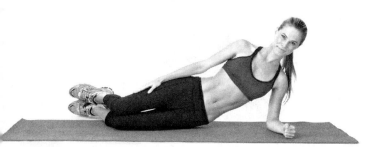 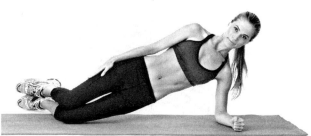

START POSITION

LEAN on your side with your forearm on the mat and your elbow directly under your shoulder. Stack your legs, knees, ankles, and feet. Bend your knees slightly. Place your other arm on your body.

THE MOVEMENT

PUSH your forearm down into the floor as you squeeze your glutes and lift your hips into the air.

YOUR weight should be on your forearm and knees and your body should be in a straight line from knees to shoulders.

HOLD at the top of the movement, then lower to the start position.

REPEAT to complete the set.

TIPS

KEEP your body in a straight line from knees to shoulders.

TIGHTEN your core muscles throughout the exercise.

C2: 45° Back Extension

LOCATION: GYM

This exercise targets the muscles along the spine (erector spinae) well as your glutes and hamstrings.

Sets: 3
Reps: 10 to 12
Load: To be determined
Tempo: 2-0-1-1
Rest interval: 45 seconds

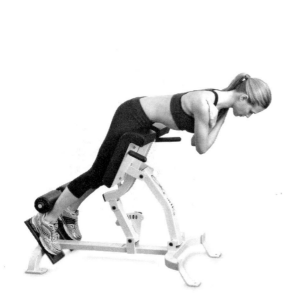

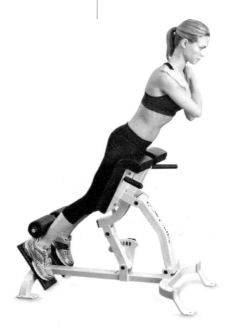

START POSITION

POSITION your thighs on the padded rests. Place your heels on the platform or under the brace.

CROSS your arms over your chest. Lean over so that your body forms a 90° angle and your torso is parallel to the floor.

THE MOVEMENT

CONTRACT your glutes and lower-back muscles and raise your torso until your body forms a straight line from ankles to shoulders.

RETURN to the start position and repeat to complete the set.

TIPS

AS you raise up, make sure your shoulders are down and that you're squeezing your shoulder blades together.

KEEP your head and spine in proper alignment.

IF you need added resistance, hold a plate or dumbbell across your chest.

C2: Swiss Ball Back Extension

LOCATION: HOME

This exercise targets the muscles along the spine (erector spinae), as well as your glutes and hamstrings.

Sets: 3
Reps: 10 to 12
Load: To be determined
Tempo: 2-0-1-1
Rest interval: 45 seconds

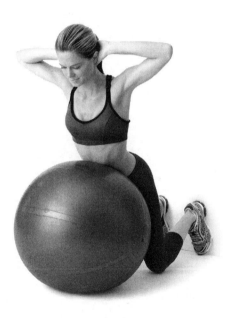

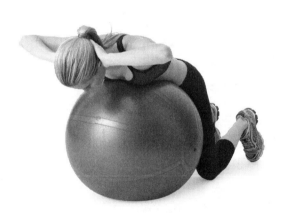

START POSITION

LIE near a wall with your abdomen and thighs on the stability ball; your body should form a 45° angle to the floor. Brace your feet against the wall; pull your toes to your shins. Touch your fingertips just behind your ears and flare your elbows out. Balance on the tips of your toes.

THE MOVEMENT

RAISE your body slowly, using your lower back. Think about raising one vertebra at a time, so that you finish with your torso at a 45° angle to the floor.

INTERMEDIATE/ADVANCED: For each rep, hold for up to a count of 3 at the top of the movement.

RETURN to the start position.

REPEAT to complete set.

TIPS

AS you raise up, make sure your shoulders are down and that you're squeezing your shoulder blades together.

KEEP your head and spine in proper alignment.

INTERMEDIATE/ADVANCED: To make the exercise more challenging, extend your arms in a Y position and maintain this position through-out the movement.

PHASE 2 STRENGTH-TRAINING PROGRAM B

Dynamic Warmup

Perform the Dynamic Warmup in Program A.

Activation Drills

	Sets	Reps	Load	Tempo	Rest	Intensity
A: Supine Glute Bridge with Medicine Ball	1	10–12	TBD	2-0-1-1	—	Low
B: Floor Y	1	6	b/w	2-0-1-1	30 sec	Low

Strength Training

	Sets	Reps	Load	Tempo	Rest
A1: Plié Squat	3	10–12	TBD	3-0-1-0	45 sec
A2: Incline Dumbbell Bench Press	3	10–12	TBD	3-0-1-0	45 sec
B1: Romanian Deadlift with Dumbbells	3	10–12	TBD	3-0-1-0	45 sec
B2: Standing Straight-Arm Cable Pulldown	3	10–12	TBD	3-0-1-0	45 sec
C1: Seated Dumbbell Curl to Military Press	3	10–12	TBD	2-0-2-0	45 sec
C2: Oblique Crunch	3	10–12/side	b/w	2-0-2-0	45 sec

Dynamic Warmup

PERFORM the warmup in Program A.

Activation Drills

A: Supine Glute Bridge with Medicine Ball*

LOCATION: HOME OR GYM

This exercise activates the hamstrings, glutes, adductors, and muscles of the lower back.

Sets: 1

Reps: 10 to 12

Load: 2- to 3-pound medicine ball

Tempo: 2-0-1-1

Rest interval: —

Intensity: Low

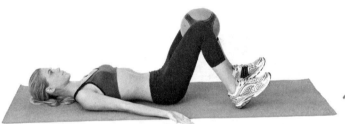

START POSITION

LIE on your back with your feet flat on the floor. Place a medicine ball between your knees and squeeze. Pull your toes up toward your shins.

PLACE your arms at your sides, with your palms facing the ceiling.

THE MOVEMENT

TIGHTEN your glutes, press against the ball, and raise your hips up off the floor. Hold for at least 1 count.

RETURN to the start position.

TIPS

KEEP your toes pulled toward your shins throughout the exercise.

MAKE sure you press down through your heels while trying to extend your knees away from your hips.

AT the top of the movement, your knees, hips, and shoulders should form a straight line.

*Home user can place a rolled-up towel between the knees if no medicine ball is available.

B: Floor Y

LOCATION: HOME OR GYM

This exercise activates the upper-back musculature, particularly the lower trapezius and the muscles in the back of the shoulder (posterior deltoids).

Sets: 1
Reps: 6
Load: Body weight
Tempo: 2-0-1-1
Rest interval: 30 seconds
Intensity: Low

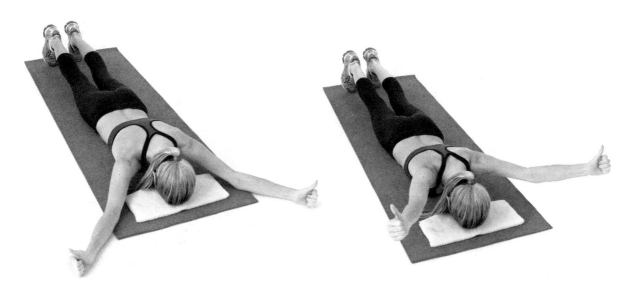

START POSITION

LIE on your stomach, resting your forehead on a towel. Draw your feet in so your toes are on the floor.

BRING your hands up over your head at a 45° angle, thumbs facing the ceiling. If someone was looking down at your position, your arms would form the letter Y.

THE MOVEMENT

FROM the start position, raise your arms up toward the ceiling. Hold.

LOWER your arms to the start position, always keeping your thumbs toward the ceiling.

REPEAT to complete the set.

TIPS

MAINTAIN the Y position throughout the exercise.

KEEP your neck long and your shoulders down.

FOCUS on bringing your shoulder blades down and in toward the spine.

Strength Training

A1: Plié Squat

LOCATION: HOME OR GYM

This exercise targets the quadriceps, hamstrings, adductors, and glutes.

Sets: 3	
Reps: 10 to 12	
Load: To be determined	
Tempo: 3-0-1-0	
Rest interval: 45 seconds	

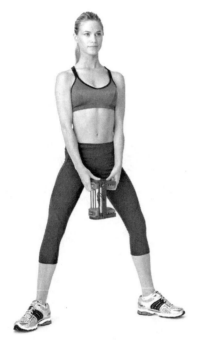

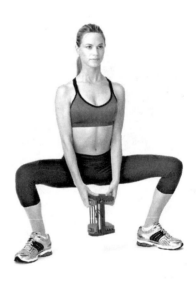

START POSITION

HOLDING a dumbbell in front of you, stand with your feet slightly more than shoulder-width apart. Keep your spine straight, chest up, and shoulders down. Turn out your toes and knees in a comfortable position. Align your knees with your toes throughout the exercise.

THE MOVEMENT

BEND your knees, lowering your hips into a squat position so that your thighs are parallel or slightly above parallel to the floor. Keep your abdominals tight and do not round your lower back.

RETURN to the start position and repeat to complete the set.

TIPS

SQUAT slowly until your thighs are almost parallel to ground.

KEEP your shoulder blades drawn back throughout the movement.

AS you rise, push down through your heels.

A2: Incline Dumbbell Bench Press

LOCATION: HOME OR GYM

This exercise targets the upper chest muscles, shoulders, and triceps.

Sets: 3

Reps: 10 to 12

Load: To be determined

Tempo: 3-0-1-0

Rest interval: 45 seconds

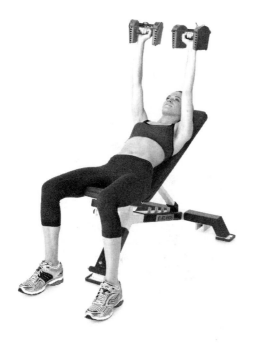
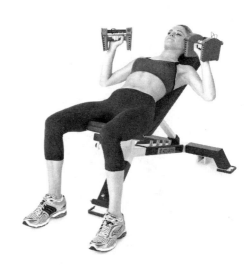

START POSITION

SET an incline bench to a 30° angle and set the dumbbells on the end. Pick up the dumbbells and sit on the bench; set the ends of the weights on your knees.

LEAN back onto the bench, using your legs to help push the dumbbells up and above your head. Your arms should be fully extended above your shoulders.

THE MOVEMENT

SLOWLY lower the dumbbells, keeping your arms at a 45° angle to your torso. Continue to lower until your upper arms are slightly below shoulder level. Keep your elbows close to your body.

RAISE the dumbbells back up without locking your elbows out at the top of the exercise.

REPEAT to complete the set.

TIPS

RAISE and lower the dumbbells with control. Do not bang them together at the top of the movement.

AT the top of the movement, keep your elbows soft, rather than locked.

B1: Romanian Deadlift with Dumbbells

LOCATION: HOME OR GYM

This exercise targets the glutes, hamstrings, and lower back.

Sets: 3
Reps: 10 to 12
Load: To be determined
Tempo: 3-0-1-0
Rest interval: 45 seconds

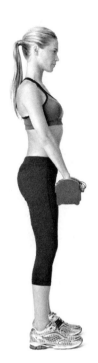

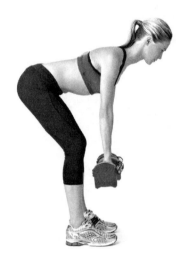

START POSITION

STAND with your feet shoulder-width apart and holding dumbbells in front of you.

THE MOVEMENT

START the movement with a slight bend in your knees.

PUSH your hips back as far as you can while bending forward at the hips and arching your lower back. Continue to bend your knees until there's about a 15° to 20° bend; you should feel a significant stretch in your hamstrings at the bottom of the movement.

TRY to keep the dumbbells as close to your legs as possible throughout the movement.

DON'T round your back during the movement.

REVERSE the movement by squeezing the glutes and extending the hips forward until you return to the start position.

REPEAT to complete the set.

TIPS

KEEP your eyes up at all times. If you look at the floor, the tendency is to round your back.

THROUGHOUT the set, keep the dumbbells as close to your body as possible.

FOCUS on lengthening your hamstrings as you lower the dumbbells and on contracting them, as well as your glutes, as you raise back up.

KEEP your shoulder blades together throughout the movement.

B2: Standing Straight-Arm Cable Pulldown

LOCATION: GYM

This exercise targets the lats and the lower trapezius muscles.

Sets: 3

Reps: 10 to 12

Load: To be determined

Tempo: 3-0-1-0

Rest interval: 45 seconds

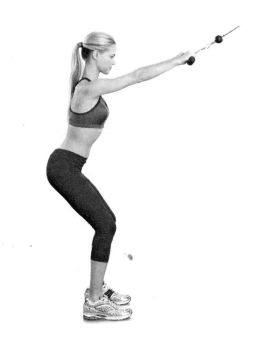
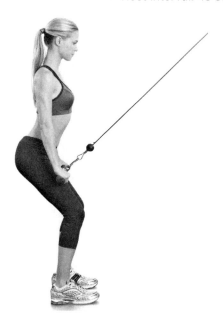

START POSITION

STAND in front of a high pulley machine; select the appropriate weight. Reach up and grasp the bar with your palms facing down, then step back slightly from the machine.

STAND with your knees slightly bent and your feet shoulder-width apart. Angle your torso forward about 30° while maintaining proper spinal alignment.

THE MOVEMENT

CONTRACT your lats and pull the bar down toward your thighs.

TRY to pull the bar as close to your thighs as you can. Imagine that invisible hands are under your upper arms and you're pressing down and in against them. Press down and in throughout the downward phase.

SLOWLY return to the start position.

REPEAT to complete the set.

TIPS

KEEP your spine straight, chest lifted, and shoulders down.

KEEP your wrists locked.

DON'T round your upper back during the movement.

B2: Standing Straight-Arm Pulldown with Tubing

LOCATION: HOME

This exercise targets the lats and the lower trapezius muscles.

Sets: 3

Reps: 10 to 12

Load: To be determined

Tempo: 3-0-1-0

Rest interval: 45 seconds

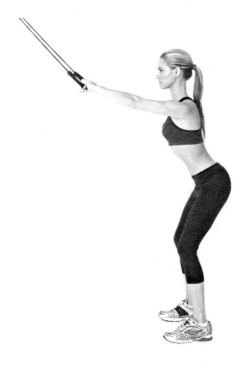
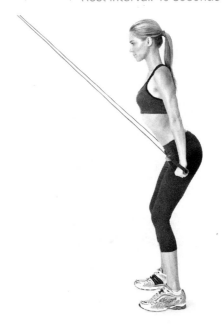

START POSITION

LOOP one end of the tubing over the top of a door. Tug a few times to ensure that the tubing is securely fastened.

GRASP the handles with your arms slightly bent.

STAND with your feet shoulder-width apart, knees slightly bent. Angle your torso slightly forward, maintaining proper spinal alignment.

THE MOVEMENT

CONTRACT your lats and pull the tubing toward your thighs. Keeping your elbows slightly bent, brace your upper body and pull the tubing until it reaches the sides of your upper thighs.

RETURN to the start position.

REPEAT to complete the set.

TIPS

KEEP your spine straight, chest lifted, and shoulders down.

KEEP your wrists locked.

DON'T round your upper back during the movement.

C1: Seated Dumbbell Curl to Military Press

LOCATION: HOME OR GYM

This movement targets the biceps and deltoids.

Sets: 3

Reps: 10 to 12

Load: To be determined

Tempo: 2-0-2-0

Rest interval: 45 seconds

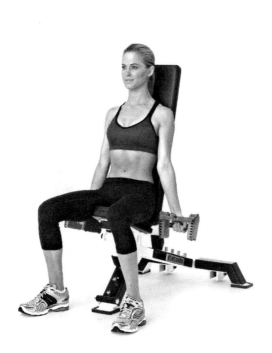 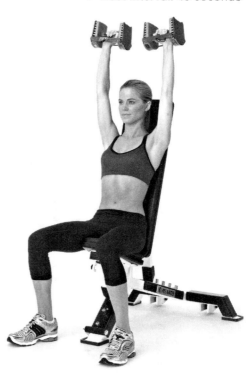

START POSITION

SIT on a bench holding dumbbells at your sides, with your feet flat on the floor.

KEEP your spine straight, chest up, and shoulders down.

THE MOVEMENT

PERFORM a dumbbell curl until the weights are at shoulder level.

ROTATING your palms so that they face away from you, press the dumbbells over the tops of your shoulders.

LOWER the weights slowly to shoulder level, then rotate palms to face toward you and return to the start position.

REPEAT to complete the set.

TIPS

CONTRACT your abdominal muscles throughout the movement.

KEEP your back straight as you perform the overhead press.

C2: Oblique Crunch

LOCATION: HOME OR GYM

This exercise targets the internal and external obliques.

Sets: 3

Reps: 10 to 12 per side

Load: Body weight

Tempo: 2-0-2-0

Rest interval: 45 seconds after completing both sides

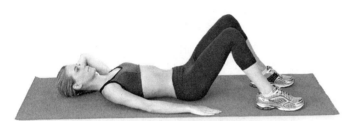 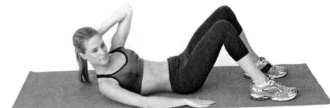

START POSITION

LIE on your back with your knees bent, feet flat on the floor, your left hand behind your head, and your left elbow open to the side. Your right arm remains flat on the floor beside you. Position your knees and feet about 6 inches apart.

THE MOVEMENT

EXHALE and lift your left shoulder to your right knee.

INHALE as you lower your shoulder.

EXHALE and lift your right shoulder to your left knee.

PERFORM all reps on one side and then repeat on the opposite side.

TIPS

THROUGHOUT this exercise, keep your elbow open to the side, rather than crunched around your head.

CRADLE your head in your fingers, and don't pull on your head.

DON'T use your hands or arms to yank your shoulder to the opposite knee.

Energy System Training: Stationary Bike

For EST workouts, use a stationary bike, preferably a Spinning bike. **For work intervals:** Increase the resistance to a level that corresponds to the prescribed RPE and heart-rate zone. Stand so your bottom is off the seat (pretend you're riding up a hill). **For recovery intervals:** Sit back down on the seat and lower the resistance to a level that corresponds to the prescribed RPE and heart-rate zone. Pedal for the duration of the recovery interval. Repeat the process for the prescribed number of intervals.

WEEK 1 (21 TO 24 MINUTES TOTAL), EST-5

WARMUP: 3 minutes, TBD; start low and build up each minute

WORKOUT: 60 seconds of work (zones 3 to 4, RPE 5 to 8), followed by 120 seconds of recovery (stationary bike: zones 1 to 2, RPE 1 to 2); repeat 5 or 6 times

COOLDOWN: 3 minutes, TBD; very low intensity

WEEK 2 (24 TO 27 MINUTES TOTAL), EST-6

WARMUP: 3 minutes, TBD; start low and build up each minute

WORKOUT: 60 seconds of work (zones 3 to 4, RPE 5 to 8), followed by 120 seconds of recovery (stationary bike: zones 1 to 2, RPE 1 to 4); repeat 6 or 7 times

COOLDOWN: 3 minutes, TBD; very low intensity

WEEK 3 (19.5 TO 22 MINUTES TOTAL), EST-7

WARMUP: 3 minutes, TBD; start low and build up each minute

WORKOUT: 45 seconds of work (zone 4, RPE 7 to 8), followed by 90 seconds of recovery (stationary bike: zones 1 to 2, RPE 1 to 4); repeat 6 or 7 times

COOLDOWN: 3 minutes, TBD; very low intensity

WEEK 4 (22 TO 26 MINUTES TOTAL), EST-8

WARMUP: 3 minutes, TBD; start low and build up each minute

WORKOUT: 30 seconds of work (zones 4 to 5, RPE 7 to 9+), followed by 90 seconds of recovery (stationary bike: zones 1 to 2, RPE 1 to 4); repeat 8 to 10 times

COOLDOWN: 3 minutes, TBD; very low intensity

EST RECOVERY SESSION (30 TO 45 MINUTES TOTAL)

WARMUP: 3 minutes, TBD; start low and build up each minute

WORKOUT: 30 to 45 minutes (zone 2, RPE 3 to 4)

COOLDOWN: 3 minutes, TBD; very low intensity

ENERGY SYSTEM TRAINING POST-WORKOUT

FOAM rolling sequence (pages 42 to 45)

STATIC stretching (pages 45 to 47)

PHASE 2 NUTRITION

Phase 2 at a Glance

> **WEEKS 1 THROUGH 4**
>
> - Bust insulin at breakfast.
> - Go crazy for cocoa.
> - Manage insulin at every meal.
> - Go on cortisol patrol.
> - Add Phase 2 supplements.

Get ready to lose the love handles and banish the back fat—or at least shrink them considerably. In Phase 2, you'll regain control of insulin and cortisol, which encourage the storage of fat, particularly in the midsection. In fact, these hormones are the main cause of that extra layer of fat that pads you from belly to bra line.

Fortunately, the right nutrition and supplementation can help rebalance these hormones. By the end of this phase, you'll have boosted your body's ability to burn fat. You'll also be more insulin sensitive, which means you'll experience fewer cravings. And if you've been diagnosed with insulin resistance, this phase will set you on the path to reversing it.

Review the sections on insulin and cortisol in Chapter 5. Then set your sights on a flatter belly, a slimmer waistline, and a sleeker bra line.

MANAGE INSULIN AT EVERY MEAL

To control insulin, the Ultimate You plan is high in fiber and protein and lower in saturated fat and simple carbohydrates. *Note*: If you are insulin resistant, follow the low-insulin protocol throughout the next three phases; see the Appendix (page 275) for more meal ideas. If you are not insulin resistant, you can opt to keep insulin low in the morning by using the low-carb breakfasts on page 166, but it is not mandatory.

- Well-timed meals keep insulin and cortisol in check. Eat every 3 to 4 hours— 3 meals and 2 snacks. Count your Recovery Shake as a snack.

- Avoid all simple, refined carbs, such as breads, pasta, and sweets.
- Use dairy sparingly. Better yet, avoid it altogether. Because dairy causes an exaggerated insulin response, it's best to avoid it if you are insulin resistant.
- Use "bites" to manage your high-fiber carb intake. If you answered yes to any of the questions on page 54, start with 4 bites of carbohydrates (about ⅓ cup) for lunch and dinner. If you answered no to most of the questions, you may have 6 bites of carbs (about ½ cup).
- You are most insulin sensitive after a workout. If you are insulin resistant, have your high-fiber carbs in your post-workout meal only, in addition to the fruit in your Recovery Shake.
- If you take 4 to 6 bites and feel lethargic or experience excessive carb cravings, switch to 6 to 8 bites. Each week, try to gradually decrease to 4 to

bust insulin at breakfast

Try these tasty, high-protein, low-carb breakfasts that keep insulin low in the morning—setting you up to burn more fat all day. They're also high in amino acids like tyrosine, which boosts your mood and enhances the brain chemicals that help you feel good and think clearly.

- **Stuffed Bell Pepper with Eggs and Avocado:** Scramble 3 eggs or 5 egg whites or 3 egg whites and 1 egg; season with sea salt and pepper, or try a dash of cayenne or chipotle pepper for a kick. Stuff into clean whole bell pepper (stem removed) and eat like a sandwich. Serve with ½ avocado, sliced.

- **Easy Eggs:** Take any scramble or omelet recipe from the Recipe Appendix (no cheese) and add a small handful of nuts; you can also try 3 eggs with 2 tablespoons fresh salsa and ½ avocado.

- **Smoked Salmon:** Have 6 ounces of smoked salmon and 1 cup of sliced cucumbers.

- **Bison Burger:** Add a small handful of nuts, plus steamed broccoli, asparagus, or a small green salad.

- **Lemon Chicken Salad:** Toss together 1 diced chicken breast, ½ cup chopped celery, and ¼ cup almonds or walnuts. Drizzle with 1 teaspoon of olive or walnut oil and 1 teaspoon of lemon juice; season with sea salt and pepper.

go crazy for cocoa

Dark cocoa and chocolate contain compounds called flavonoids that lower blood pressure, make blood less sticky, and improve insulin sensitivity. Cocoa also boosts brain chemistry in our pleasure centers, which dampens cravings for fat and sugar.

On the Ultimate You plan, you can enjoy 2 ounces of dark chocolate a day (choose an organic variety that contains at least 70 percent cocoa). Or try some of these other healthy ways to enjoy the benefits of chocolate.

Ultimate You Cocoa

- 1 tablespoon organic unsweetened cocoa powder
- 1 teaspoon xylitol or Truvia (less or more, to desired sweetness)
- ¼ teaspoon or a sprinkle of cinnamon or a dash of cayenne (optional)

Place all ingredients in mug; fill with boiling water and stir. For creamier cocoa: Fill half of the cup with hot water and the rest with unsweetened vanilla or chocolate almond milk. For chocolate soda: Prepare ½ cup cocoa as above; let cool and pour over ice. Fill rest of glass with plain seltzer.

PBJ Cocoa Meal Replacement Shake

(Use this shake as a meal replacement only.)

- 1 to ½ scoops whey powder (recommended brands: Ultimate Chocolate Whey from Hardware, Jay Robb Chocolate Whey) plus 1 to 2 teaspoons organic unsweetened cocoa powder
- ½ cup frozen cherries
- 1 tablespoon organic unsweetened peanut butter
- 1 tablespoon Ultimate Fiber (Hardware)
- ¼ cup water or coconut water
- ¼ cup unsweetened chocolate almond milk
- 1 teaspoon xylitol or erythritol, if desired

Cocoa Banana Recovery Shake

(Use this shake post-workout only.)

- 1 to 1½ scoops protein powder and 1 to 2 teaspoons organic plain cocoa powder
- 1 teaspoon honey
- ½ banana
- Ice and water or coconut water

Numi Chocolate Puerh Tea

Add a splash of unsweetened almond milk or So Delicious brand coconut milk and a bit of xylitol or erythritol to the Chocolate Puerh tea from Numi and you have an afternoon treat or a perfect way to start your day. You'll find the tea in health-food stores, or order online at www.numitea.com.

6 bites and see how you feel (use your cravings as a guide). Ultimately, insulin resistance will respond best to 4 bites of high-fiber starches only. If you're having trouble decreasing your carb intake, consult a nutritional medicine practitioner about insulin resistance. You might also take supplements that enhance insulin sensitivity (more on that in a moment), and follow the tips below.

- Add lemon or lime to your water with a meal, or take a tablespoon of vinegar before meals. This will lower the insulin response of the food. Or eat a green salad dressed with vinegar before the rest of your meal—this will moderately lower your insulin response.

- From 15 to 30 minutes before a meal, stir 1 teaspoon of a non-grain-based fiber in a glass of water and drink. See page 66 for recommended fiber brands.

GO ON CORTISOL PATROL

Managing stress is easier said than done, but you absolutely need to do it. Practice at least the basics of stress management.

- **Eat regularly.** That's right: every 3 to 4 hours. And no matter what, never skip breakfast, which raises cortisol too much and encourages fat storage. If you must schedule meals like appointments, do it, until regular mealtimes become second nature.

- **Exercise in the morning, if possible.** You'll avoid raising cortisol in the evening, when you want to wind down. You'll also be sure to get your workout in—before you have a chance to postpone it—so you'll burn more fat all day.

- **Prioritize.** Some days you can't do it all. Do what you can at work. Get to the gym. Eat healthy. Get your zzz's.

- **Take a brisk walk if you get stressed.** You'll burn off the sugar and fat liberated by the rise in cortisol and adrenaline.

- **Get your R&R.** Do not skimp on the recovery and regeneration practices in Chapter 4.

let cortisol help you burn fat

Despite its rep as the belly-fat hormone, the one time cortisol can actually help you *burn* body fat is during exercise. That's when cortisol (along with lactic acid, glucagon, and growth hormone) stimulates the liver to break down its store of sugar and break down the fat in adipose (body fat) tissue during intense exercise. Here are four ways to get this beneficial, controlled cortisol response during and after your workouts.

1. **Fuel for fat burning.** The perfect time to do high-intensity exercise is about 2 hours after a meal. Wait longer than that, and you might run out of steam; any sooner than that, and you'll be burning off your meal rather than using cortisol to dip into stored fat. If you really need to fuel up before a session, use this recipe: Mix ½ to 1 scoop whey protein with ½ cup plain water or coconut water, blend, and drink at least 1 hour before your workout. It's optimal to do less intense exercise, such as the long walks we recommend in Phase 3, on an empty stomach. *Note:* This advice is for fat loss. If your goals are athletic performance or endurance, it's vital to fuel before exercise.

2. **Train hard, not long.** Heavy weights and high-intensity sprints create the right hormonal environment to burn fat.

3. **Hydrate correctly.** Drink plain water or a sugar-free electrolyte beverage, such as Ultimate Electrolytes (Hardware) or Electrolyte Synergy (Designs for Health). Avoid sugary sports drinks that contain high-fructose corn syrup or crystalline fructose.

4. **Soup up your Recovery Shake.** To increase its effectiveness, mix in 5 to 10 grams of L-glutamine.

- **Snooze.** If you can't sleep well on your own, and if over-the-counter natural methods don't help, speak to your doctor about options.

- **Be a (dark) chocoholic.** Does it get any better? Enjoy 2 ounces of dark chocolate per day, or see page 167 for other yummy ways to enjoy cocoa.

- **If you need support, ask for it.** Get support from friends and family. Seek the help of a therapist. Schedule an appointment with a nutritional medicine practitioner, who can help balance your stress chemistry or evaluate your adrenal glands (if you've been under prolonged stress).

ADD PHASE 2 SUPPLEMENTS

Add the supplements below to the Phase 1 supplements. While the food on this plan provides many of these nutrients, research shows that supplementation may result in additional benefits. If you are insulin resistant, this protocol will dramatically improve your results. If you choose individual herbs, pick 2 or 3 or, for convenience, use a combination product.

TO CONTROL INSULIN AND BLOOD SUGAR

Herbs

Take daily as directed on the label, or in the doses below.

- Banaba leaf, 400 milligrams
- Bitter gourd (a.k.a. bitter melon), 200 milligrams
- Cinnamon, 400 milligrams
- Fenugreek, 500 milligrams
- Grapeseed extract, 200 milligrams standardized proanthocyanidins
- Green tea, 300 milligrams standardized EGCG
- Gymnema sylvestre, 200 milligrams
- And don't forget your non-grain-based fiber supplement: 1 tablespoon, 1 to 5 times daily.

Nutrients

Find a multivitamin that contains chromium, magnesium, vanadyl sulfate, taurine, and L-carnitine. Ultimate Metabolic Multi (Hardware) contains these nutrients as well as some of the herbs above. Take 2 Ultimate Metabolic Multis with each meal (6 per day). Take other multivitamins as directed on the label.

Also include:

- CLA: Research has shown that 2 to 6 grams per day can improve insulin sensitivity and reduce belly fat. Take 2 grams 3 times daily with meals. We recommend Clarinol. This patented form of CLA contains the type of CLA associated with fat loss. Visit www.clarinol.com, or try Ultimate CLA (Hardware).

- R-lipoic acid: Research shows that 600 to 1,000 milligrams per day improves insulin sensitivity. Ensure that the brand you buy is not a blend of R and S forms—opt for R form only. Ultimate Metabolic Multi contains 600 milligrams stabilized R-lipoic acid.

Foods

- Grass-fed beef and bison: They're high in CLA, taurine, carnitine, and magnesium.

- Green tea: Drink a few cups each day.

- Cinnamon: Sprinkle at least ¼ teaspoon in a cup of coffee or tea, or mix it into protein shakes or on your high-fiber carbs.

TO MANAGE CORTISOL

Herbs

Take daily as directed on the label, or in the doses below.

- Coleus forskohlii, 250 milligrams standardized to at least 10 percent forskohlii, twice daily

- Rhodiola, 100 milligrams

- Licorice, 20 milligrams

- Holy basil, 400 milligrams

- American ginseng, 100 milligrams

- Green tea, 300 milligrams standardized EGCG

Note: If possible, take first thing in the morning and at lunchtime or mid-afternoon; herbs that support adrenal balance often work best at these times.

Cautions

- Avoid licorice if you have high blood pressure.

- EGCG extracts often contain caffeine, so take them earlier in the day.

NUTRIENTS

Take daily as directed on the label, or in the doses below.

- Phosphatidyl serine (PS) boosts memory and protects against the damaging effects of stress. Take 300 to 400 milligrams at dinner and at bedtime. Or use ½ teaspoon of the topical cream Adrenacalm, available at www. bodybyhardware.com.

how to beat the bloat

Your body holds extra water for many reasons, including hormonal changes during PMS, lack of sleep, high stress, and dehydration, often from alcohol or as a result of several days of low water intake. Even flying can cause puffiness! Also, if you're on a lower-carb diet plan, a day or so of higher carb intake will puff you up (those carbs boost your body's store of glycogen).

Happily, there are ways to shed the water to look and feel leaner and to avoid the puffiness in the first place. Here's how.

To shed water weight:

- **Take taurine.** This amino acid is a natural diuretic. Take 2 grams twice daily for 1 week (consider Water Ease by Designs for Health). *Note: Taurine will lower blood pressure due to its diuretic action. Avoid if you have low blood pressure or adrenal insufficiency (i.e., Addison's disease), unless supervised.*

- **Load up on green veggies.** Asparagus and celery are natural diuretics. Lettuce, cucumbers, and kale are good, too.

- **Avoid dairy and wheat entirely.** These foods tend to be inflammatory in most people, leading to more puffiness.

- **Manage your carbs.** Eat no more than 4 to 6 bites per meal, opting for higher-fiber options, such as root veggies and fruit.

- **Return to recommended water intake.** If you've been slacking, get your fill (see formula on page 73 to determine your recommended intake).

To prevent water weight:

- **Keep water intake steady.** Avoid days of low intake—if you are dehydrated, you'll hold water when you start drinking more.

- **When you drink, hydrate.** Alcohol acts as a diuretic, making you lose excess water. This loss quickly leads to dehydration, causing the body to preserve the water you drink—particularly the next morning. Drink one glass of water for every alcoholic beverage to avoid dehydration.

- **Don't forget your supplements.** Keep your cells healthy with minerals found in a good multivitamin and in high-quality omega-3 fatty acids.

- Magnesium and taurine support cortisol and insulin. Take 600 to 1,000 milligrams in divided doses of magnesium glycinate and 1 to 2 grams taurine 2 or 3 times daily. For a taurine supplement, consider Water Ease from Designs for Health, and take 2 capsules twice daily.

Cautions

- High doses of magnesium may cause loose stools. If this happens to you, try a topical magnesium, such as MagneDerm (Designs for Health) or Topical Mag (Poliquin Performance).

For ease and to decrease your overall capsule intake, try this combo regimen.

- Ultimate Metabolic Multi: 2 capsules with each meal
- Ultimate CLA: 2 capsules with each meal
- Ultimate Fat Burner: 1 to 3 capsules with each meal. This formula contains EGCG, Banaba, green tea, garcinia, American ginseng, chromium, vanadyl sulfate, magnesium, and coleus.
- Ultimate Insulin Manager: Start with 1 to 3 capsules with each meal and snack; if you are still feeling sleepy after eating, increase dosage by 1 capsule until you no longer have any postmeal fatigue—this is your ongoing dose. This formula contains fenugreek, cinnamon, gymnema, Banaba, and other ingredients.

CHAPTER 10

Phase 3: Intensification

GET READY FOR SOME BIG changes in Phase 3. If you've followed the first 2 phases faithfully, you should be ready for the challenge.

ULTIMATE YOU WORKOUT

Our goals are to continue to increase lean muscle mass, decrease body fat, and begin using mini-circuits during the strength-training sessions.

You'll train 6 times a week—3 strength-training sessions, 2 EST sessions, and 1 EST recovery session. As in Phase 1, you can train at the gym or at home. Here's the run-down on your Phase 3 workout.

- STRENGTH TRAINING: As in Phase 2, you will alternate between two different strength-training programs: A and B. Each week, one of the programs will get a higher priority, and you will perform it twice that week. As in Phases 1 and 2, always perform the dynamic warmup and the activation drills.

  While the dynamic warmup remains the same for both Programs A and B, two of the activation drills will change each workout so that you can target different areas.

  In the strength-training portion, you will perform mini-circuits of three exercises. One of the exercises in the mini-circuit will be a calisthenic exercise. These mini-circuits are designed so that you do more work in a given period of time.

- EST: In this phase, we will continue to perform anaerobic interval training, but you will use a treadmill, or you can walk and run outside.

The anaerobic interval sessions should take anywhere from 23½ to 28 minutes, including warmup and cooldown. Please remember to use your unique heart-rate and RPE training zones. These workouts will intensify each week, which will ultimately help you get leaner. You'll also perform a weekly EST recovery workout—36 to 55 minutes (including warmup and cooldown) of a low-intensity steady-state cardio session, such as a brisk walk or slow jog.

- RECOVERY: Always foam roll after each workout in both your EST and resistance-training sessions. Perform static stretching after each EST session, and feel free to do it after resistance-training sessions, too (after you've foam rolled). You can also perform foam rolling before the dynamic warmup of the resistance-training session, particularly if you're feeling sore or tight. And feel free to incorporate some other recovery techniques from Chapter 4 as well. Remember: Muscles repair, rebuild, and strengthen when you rest, not when you train.

ULTIMATE YOU NUTRITION

Rev Up Your Lean Hormones; Reset Your Female Hormones

In Phase 3, you'll rev up fat-burning testosterone and growth hormone with intense workouts and adequate sleep and dietary protein. You'll also identify and treat hormone-based health issues, including menstrual irregularities, PMS symptoms, and menopausal hot flashes.

Lower Your Estrogen Burden

We'll make the case for going hard-core organic—including switching over to all-natural body-care products and cosmetics and rethinking hormonal birth control and synthetic hormone replacement therapy (HRT). Both will help prevent and treat a major cause of fat gain in women: estrogen dominance.

PHASE 3 WORKOUT AT A GLANCE

We've designed 2 separate strength-training routines for this phase: Programs A and B. For the next 4 weeks, you will alternate between them.

The EST sessions will be different each week, with the exception of the recovery session, which is the same for Phases 2 through 4.

- HOW LONG: 4 weeks
- HOW OFTEN: 6 times a week
    - 3 Phase 3 strength-training sessions
    - 2 EST sessions
    - 1 EST recovery session
- GOALS: Continue to increase lean muscle mass; continue to decrease body fat; introduce circuit weight training.

WEEK	MONDAY	TUESDAY	WEDNESDAY	THURSDAY	FRIDAY	SATURDAY	SUNDAY
1	Strength 3-A	EST-9	Strength 3-B	EST-9	Strength 3-A	EST-R	Off
2	Strength 3-B	EST-10	Strength 3-A	EST-10	Strength 3-B	EST-R	Off
3	Strength 3-A	EST-11	Strength 3-B	EST-11	Strength 3-A	EST-R	Off
4	Strength 3-B	EST-12	Strength 3-A	EST-12	Strength 3-B	EST-R	Off

PHASE 3 STRENGTH-TRAINING PROGRAM A

Dynamic Warmup

	Sets	Reps	Load	Tempo	Rest	Intensity
A: Forward Lunge with Twist	1	5/side	b/w	Slow	—	Low
B: Sumo Squat to Stand	1	4–5	b/w	Slow	30 sec	Low

Activation Drills

	Sets	Reps	Load	Tempo	Rest	Intensity
A: Mini-Band Walking—Lateral	1	10/side	TBD	Slow	—	Low
B: Standing Y, T, and W	1	4 each	b/w	Slow	30 sec	Low

Strength Training

	Sets	Reps	Load	Tempo	Rest
A1: Front Dumbbell Squat	3	8–10	TBD	3-0-1-0	Up to 10 sec
A2: Standing Cable Chest Fly	3	8–10	TBD	3-0-1-0	Up to 10 sec
A3: Low-Box Lateral Shuffle	3	30–75 sec	b/w	Mod–fast	60–90 sec
B1: Reverse Hyperextension	3	8–10	b/w	2-0-2-0	Up to 10 sec
B2: Single-Arm Dumbbell Row	3	8–10/side	TBD	2-0-1-1	—
B3: Mountain Climber	3	30–75 sec	b/w	Mod–fast	60–90 sec
C1: Lying Dumbbell Triceps Extension	3	8–10	TBD	2-1-1-0	Up to 10 sec
C2: Swiss Ball Oblique Crunch	3	8–10/side	b/w	2-0-2-0	Up to 10 sec
C3: Jumping Jacks	3	30–75/side	b/w	Mod–fast	60–90 sec

Dynamic Warmup

A: Forward Lunge with Twist

LOCATION: HOME OR GYM

This exercise warms up the hips, legs, and core.

Sets: 1	
Reps: 5 per side	
Load: Body weight	
Tempo: Slow	
Rest interval: —	
Intensity: Low	

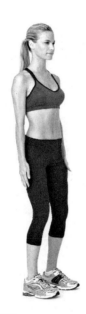
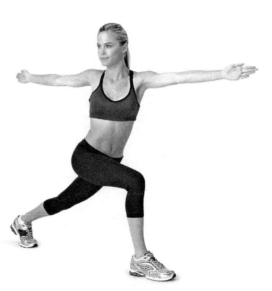

START POSITION

STAND with your feet hip-width apart, arms at your sides.

THE MOVEMENT

LUNGE forward with your right leg, bending that knee 90°.

AS you step forward into the lunge with your right foot, raise both arms in front of you to shoulder level, palms facing each other. Then, rotate right arm and torso to the right.

RETURN to the start position. Repeat movement on the left side. Perform 5 total on each side.

TIPS

STEP forward with your less-dominant leg first.

KEEP both arms raised at shoulder level as you rotate.

STEP out and rotate your torso only to your comfort level.

B: Sumo Squat to Stand

LOCATION: HOME OR GYM

This exercise elongates the hamstrings, lower back, and inner thigh muscles (adductors) and opens up the hips.

Sets: 1
Reps: 4 to 5
Load: Body weight
Tempo: Slow
Rest interval: 30 seconds
Intensity: Low

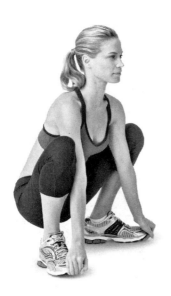

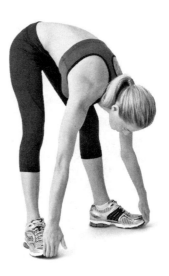

START POSITION

STAND forward, feet greater than shoulder-width apart. Turn your feet out slightly; keep your knees in the same line as your feet.

BEND your knees and drop your butt as close to your heels as possible. Reach your hands and arms inside your knees and grip the toes of your workout shoes. Keep your head and chest up.

THE MOVEMENT

BEGIN to stand, keeping your grip on your sneakers.

RISE slowly until your hips are higher than your shoulders and you are just about to lose your

fingers' grip. If possible, straighten your legs fully. If you can't get this far up without letting go of your toes, simply return to the start position.

REPEAT to complete the set.

TIPS

IN the start position, keep your head and chest lifted.

KEEP your back as flat as possible throughout the exercise. Try not to round it.

RAISE your hips only to where you can still grip your sneakers. The more flexible you are, the higher you'll be able to raise your hips.

IF you have very good range of motion, try to contract your quads as you raise up.

Activation Drills

A: Mini-Band Walking—Lateral (Program A)

LOCATION: HOME OR GYM

This exercise targets the outer hip muscles, in particular the gluteus medius.

Sets: 1
Reps: 10 per side
Load: To be determined
Tempo: Slow
Rest interval: —
Intensity: Low

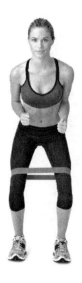 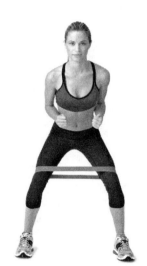 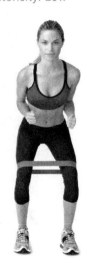

START POSITION

WRAP the mini-band around your legs, just above your knees. Stand with your feet shoulder-width apart; bend your knees slightly and lean slightly forward at the hips.

PLACE your hands on your hips or hold them directly in front of you in an athletic position.

THE MOVEMENT

STEP 8 to 10 inches out with the left leg.

SLOWLY bring your right leg in 8 to 10 inches.

REPEAT for a total of 10 steps, then switch sides and step to the right for 10 steps.

TIPS

LEAD the movement with the knee rather than the foot. Pushing outward from the knee first, rather than thinking of stepping, will engage your outer hip muscles.

MAINTAIN good spinal alignment. Do not round your lower back.

KEEP your shoulders parallel to the floor throughout the movement. Do not dip your torso to the right or left.

B: Standing Y, T, and W

LOCATION: HOME OR GYM

These exercises target the muscles of the upper back (rhomboids and trapezius) and the backs of the shoulders.

Note: For each of these three movements, make sure not to shrug your shoulders as you perform the movements. Keep your shoulders down and your neck long.

Sets: 1
Reps: 4 repetitions of each
Load: Body weight
Tempo: Slow
Rest interval: 30 seconds
Intensity: Low

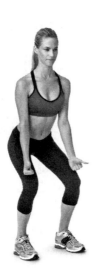

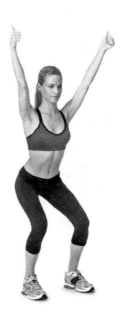

START POSITION

STAND with your feet shoulder-width apart; bend your knees slightly and lean slightly forward at the hips.

STANDING Y

WITH your hands in front of you, rotate your palms slightly out, thumbs pointing forward.

SLOWLY lift your arms so that at the top of the movement, you look like the letter Y. Focus on keeping your shoulders down and back.

RETURN to the start position and repeat to complete the set.

AFTER the fourth repetition, move into the standing T.

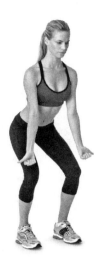
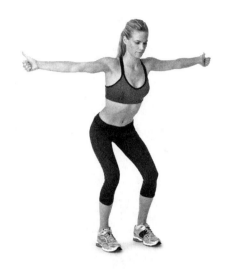

STANDING T

ROTATE your hands so that your palms face away from your body. Point your thumbs away from your midline.

SLOWLY lift your arms to shoulder height (or slightly above shoulder height, if you can) so

that at the top of the movement, you look like the letter T. Focus on bringing your shoulders together.

AFTER the fourth repetition, move into the standing W.

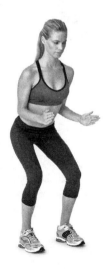
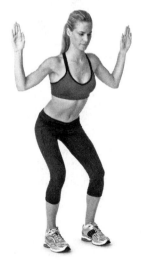

STANDING W

HOLD your hands in front of you, palms facing each other, elbows bent. Your forearms and upper arms should form an angle slightly larger than 90°.

SLOWLY lift your arms and rotate your upper arms and forearms back so that at the top of the movement, you look like the letter W. Focus on keeping your shoulders down and back.

Strength Training

A1: Front Dumbbell Squat

LOCATION: HOME OR GYM

This exercise targets the quadriceps, hamstrings, and glutes, as well as the core.

Sets: 3

Reps: 8 to 10

Tempo: 3-0-1-0

Load: To be determined

Rest Interval: Up to 10 seconds

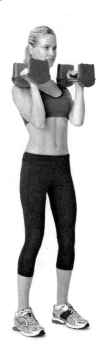

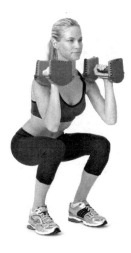

START POSITION

STAND with your feet about shoulder-width apart. Hold a pair of dumbbells with your palms facing each other, resting the dumbbells on the front of your shoulders.

THE MOVEMENT

KEEP your torso as upright as possible; lower yourself as far as you can by pushing your hips back and bending your knees.

MAINTAIN your arms in the same position throughout the entire movement.

RETURN to the start position and repeat for the prescribed number of reps.

TIP

KEEP your chest up and maintain a slight curve in your lower back throughout the movement.

A2: Standing Cable Chest Fly

LOCATION: GYM

This exercise targets the muscles of the chest.

Sets: 3

Reps: 8 to 10

Load: To be determined

Tempo: 3-0-1-0

Rest interval: Up to 10 seconds

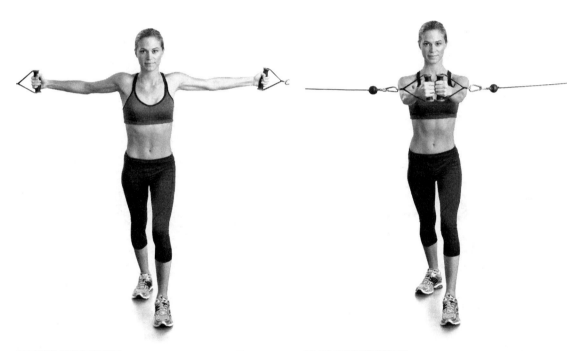

START POSITION

PLACE a single-handed connection on each of the cables, using the hook on the end of the cable. Set the proper amount of weight.

STAND between the two cables with one in each hand. Extend your arms fully and step forward with one foot. Maintain good spinal alignment.

THE MOVEMENT

BRING your hands together, palms facing each other.

RETURN to the start position. Repeat to complete the set.

TIPS

FOCUS on squeezing your chest muscles as you bring your arms together.

MAKE sure elbows stay fully extended, but not locked.

A2: Standing Cable Chest Press with Tubing

LOCATION: HOME

This exercise targets the muscles of the chest, anterior deltoids, and triceps.

Sets: 3

Reps: 8 to 10

Load: To be determined

Tempo: 3-0-1-0

Rest interval: Up to 10 seconds

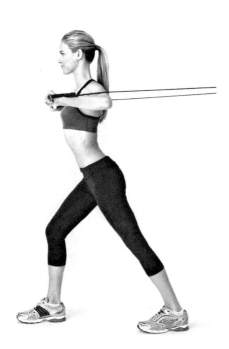 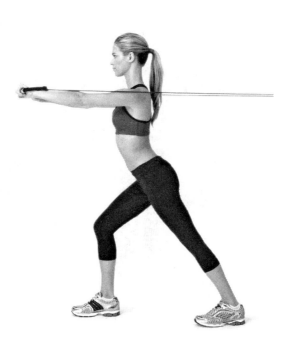

START POSITION

WRAP the tubing or band around a sturdy shoulder-height object such as a bedpost or stair railing. Grasp the tubing with your palms facing forward. Stand with one foot forward.

THE MOVEMENT

PRESS forward until your arms are fully extended in front of you. Keep your arms straight and parallel to the floor.

RETURN to the start position. Repeat to complete the set.

TIP

KEEP your core tight throughout the exercise. Focus on squeezing your chest muscles as you bring your arms forward.

A3: Low-Box Lateral Shuffle

LOCATION: HOME OR GYM

This exercise targets the strength, stability, and coordination of the entire lower body.

Sets: 3

Reps: 30 to 75 seconds

Load: Body weight

Tempo: Moderate to fast

Rest interval: 60 to 90 seconds

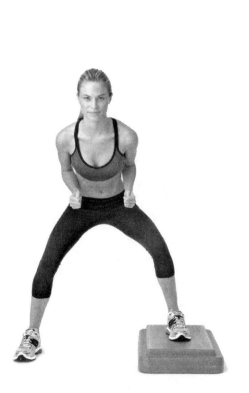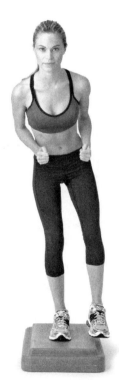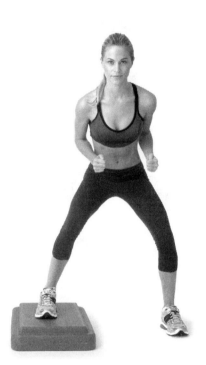

START POSITION

STAND with your left foot on the box and your right foot on the floor, about a foot away from the box.

LEAN torso forward slightly.

THE MOVEMENT

JUMP sideways so that your right foot lands on the box and your left foot on the floor.

CONTINUE to shuffle on and off the step from side to side for 30 to 75 seconds.

TIPS

FORM before speed. Master the shuffling movement before you speed up.

WHEN you have mastered the movement, attempt to increase the speed of your jumps, keeping your landings short.

B1: Reverse Hyperextension

LOCATION: GYM

This exercise targets the erector spinae, glutes, and hamstrings.

Sets: 3

Reps: 8 to 10

Load: Body weight

Tempo: 2-0-2-0

Rest interval: Up to 10 seconds

START POSITION

POSITION yourself on a 90° back-extension bench. Place your hips on the pads and hold the back of the bench (where your feet normally go).

THE MOVEMENT

SQUEEZING glutes, raise your legs until they are parallel to the floor. Keep your head in line with your spine.

LOWER your legs to the start position and repeat to complete the set.

TIPS

KEEP your feet in a neutral position (as pictured) so that the tops of your feet are 90° to your shins.

DON'T let your legs come too far forward, as you want to maintain a neutral lumbar spine (i.e., no rounding of the lower back).

B1: Reverse Hyperextension over Swiss Ball

LOCATION: HOME

This exercise targets the erector spinae, glutes, and hamstrings.

Sets: 3

Reps: 8 to 10

Load: To be determined

Tempo: 2-0-2-0

Rest interval: Up to 10 seconds

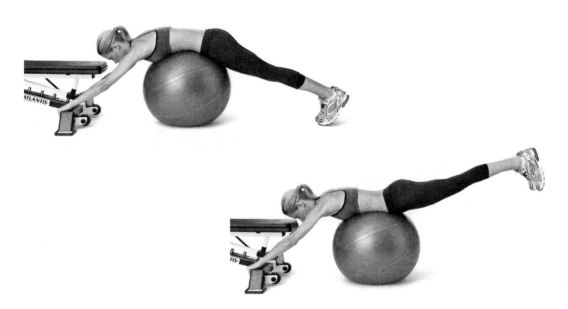

START POSITION

LIE on your stomach over a Swiss ball. Allow your legs to hang off the edge of the ball, and keep your toes on the floor.

HOLD on to a sturdy piece of gym equipment (or the legs of a sturdy table or other immovable object) for support.

THE MOVEMENT

CONTRACT your glutes and raise your legs so that your shoulders, hips, knees, and ankles form a straight line.

RETURN to the start position. Repeat to complete the set.

TIPS

KEEP your feet in a neutral position (as pictured) so that the tops of your feet are 90° to your shins.

MAKE sure you maintain a neutral lumbar spine (i.e., do not excessively arch your lower back), and keep your head in line with your spine.

B2: Single-Arm Dumbbell Row

LOCATION: HOME OR GYM

This exercise targets the lats, rhomboids, and lower and middle trapezius.

Sets: 3

Reps: 8 to 10 per side

Load: To be determined

Tempo: 2-0-1-1

Rest interval: Up to 10 seconds

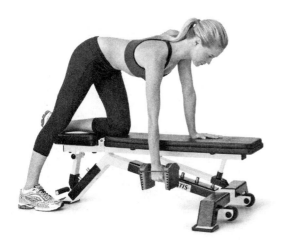 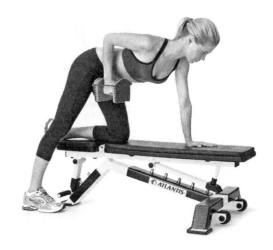

START POSITION

PLACE one hand and one knee on a flat bench.

PLACE your other foot on the floor next to the bench. Grasp the dumbbell with your free hand; extend your arm straight to the floor with your palm facing toward you.

KEEP your back straight; your torso should remain parallel to the floor.

THE MOVEMENT

BEND your elbow and lift the dumbbell to your side, keeping your elbow close to your body and your back as straight as a tabletop. At the top of the movement, make sure you draw your shoulder blade down and back.

RETURN to the start position. Repeat to complete the set.

TIPS

KEEP a small arch in your lower back.

PULL by leading with your elbow.

IF you have to jerk the dumbbell up, you're probably using too much weight.

MAINTAIN proper spinal alignment; do not round your back and do not rotate your torso.

B3: Mountain Climber

LOCATION: HOME OR GYM

This exercise targets the strength and stability of your entire body (lower extremities, core, and upper extremities).

Sets: 3

Reps: 30 to 75 seconds

Load: Body weight

Tempo: Moderate to fast

Rest interval: 60 to 90 seconds

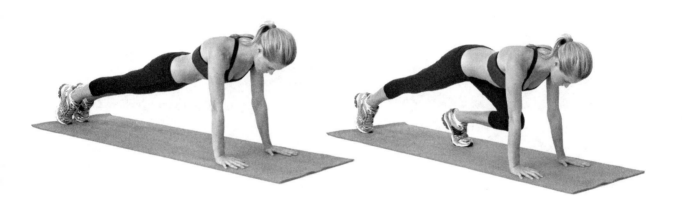

START POSITION

ASSUME a pushup position on your hands and toes, hands shoulder-with apart.

BRING one knee in toward your chest, raising your heel and resting your weight on the ball of your foot.

THE MOVEMENT

JUMP up and switch feet in the air, bringing the forward foot back and the back foot forward.

CONTINUE alternating your feet as fast as you safely can for the duration of the set.

TIPS

SLIGHTLY contract your abdominal muscles throughout the exercise.

MAKE sure your forward leg and your hands support your weight.

KEEP hips and torso parallel to the floor, and keep your head in line with your spine.

C1: Lying Dumbbell Triceps Extension

LOCATION: HOME OR GYM

This exercise targets the triceps.

Sets: 3

Reps: 8 to 10

Load: To be determined

Tempo: 2-1-1-0

Rest interval: Up to 10 seconds

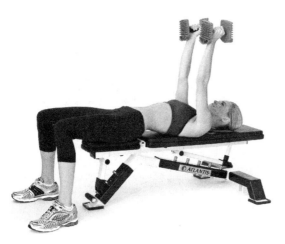
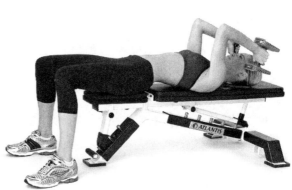

START POSITION

LIE on a flat bench with your feet flat on the floor. Hold the dumbbells straight over your shoulders.

THE MOVEMENT

KEEPING your upper arms in the same position, lower the dumbbells by bending your elbows so that forearms are slightly lower than parallel to the floor. The dumbbells will be on either side of your head.

SQUEEZE your triceps and return to the start position. Repeat to complete the set.

TIPS

DON'T use too much weight. You will not be able to maintain proper arm position during the lowering phase of the movement.

KEEP your elbows in throughout the exercise.

KEEP your upper arms still as you lower the dumbbells, being careful to prevent them from hitting your head.

C2: Swiss Ball Oblique Crunch

LOCATION: GYM OR HOME

This exercise targets the obliques.

Sets: 3

Reps: 8 to 10 per side

Load: Body weight

Tempo: 2-0-2-0

Rest interval: Up to 10 seconds

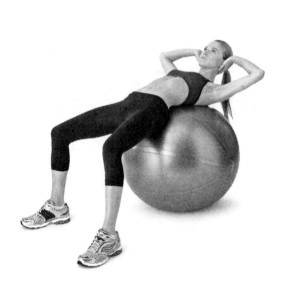 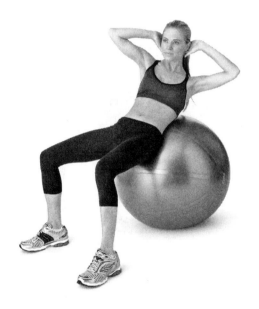

START POSITION

SIT on a stability ball with your feet flat on the floor.

WALK your feet forward as you roll your body back onto the ball until your lower back is supported by the ball.

PLACE your fingertips behind your ears. (You may also cross your arms over your chest.)

THE MOVEMENT

SLOWLY raise your torso, keeping your elbows wide and bringing your right elbow toward (but not to) your left knee.

RETURN to the start position. Repeat 8 to 10 reps on your right side. Then perform on your left side to complete the set.

TIPS

KEEP your lower back in contact with the ball and your elbows pointed outward.

DO not try to touch your elbow to your knee or pull on your neck.

C3: Jumping Jacks

LOCATION: HOME OR GYM

This exercise strengthens your entire body.

Sets: 3

Reps: 30 to 75 seconds

Load: Body weight

Tempo: Moderate to fast

Rest interval: 60 to 90 seconds

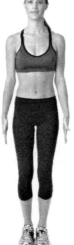

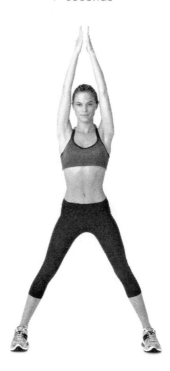

START POSITION

START with your feet a couple of inches apart and hold your hands at your sides. Keep your back straight and look straight ahead.

THE MOVEMENT

BENDING your knees slightly, jump up and spread your feet about 2 to 3 feet apart. Land on the balls of your feet before your heels touch the ground.

AT the same time, keep your arms straight and bring them up from your sides in one arc, ending with your hands together above your head.

RETURN to the start position. Repeat for the duration of the set.

TIP

WHEN you land from your jump, your feet should be 2 to 3 feet apart.

PHASE 3 STRENGTH-TRAINING PROGRAM B

Dynamic Warmup

	Sets	Reps	Load	Tempo	Rest	Intensity
A: Forward Lunge with Twist	1	5/side	b/w	Slow	—	Low
B: Sumo Squat to Stand	1	4–5	b/w	Slow	30 sec	Low

Activation Drills

	Sets	Reps	Load	Tempo	Rest	Intensity
A: Supine Glute Bridge—Marching	1	5/sec	b/w	Slow	—	Low
B: Standing Y, T, and W	1	4 each	b/w	Slow	30 sec	Low

Strength Training

	Sets	Reps	Load	Tempo	Rest
A1: Reverse Lunge	3	8–10/side	TBD	3-0-1-0	Up to 10 sec
A2: Flat Dumbbell Fly	3	8–10	TBD	3-0-1-0	Up to 10 sec
A3: Skipping Rope	3	45–120 sec	b/w	Mod–fast	60–90 sec
B1: Single-Leg Romanian Deadlift	3	8–10/side	TBD	2-1-1-0	Up to 10 sec
B2: Incline Prone Reverse Fly	3	8–10	TBD	2-0-1-1	Up to 10 sec
B3: Skipping Rope	3	45–120 sec	b/w	Mod–fast	60–90 sec
C1: Standing Dumbbell Curl	3	8–10	TBD	3-0-1-0	Up to 10 sec
C2: Prone Knee Pull-In on Swiss Ball	3	8–10	b/w	2-0-2-0	Up to 10 sec
C3: Skipping Rope	3	45–120 sec	b/w	Mod–fast	60–90 sec

Dynamic Warmup and Activation Drills

PERFORM the warmup and drills in Program A.

A: Supine Glute Bridge—Marching (Program B)

LOCATION: HOME OR GYM

This exercise activates the glutes.

Sets: 1
Reps: 5 per side
Load: Body weight
Tempo: Slow
Rest interval: —
Intensity: Low

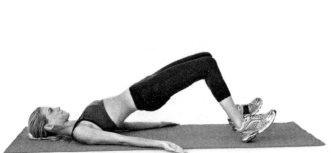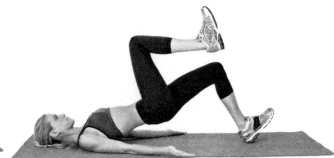

START POSITION

LIE faceup on the floor with your arms at your sides. Bend your knees and place your heels on the floor, with toes raised. Slightly contract your abdominals.

LIFT your hips off the floor until your body forms a straight line from knees to shoulders.

THE MOVEMENT

HOLDING this position, lift one knee to your chest, as if you're marching.

RETURN to the start position and "march" with the other leg.

REPEAT for the prescribed number of repetitions.

TIPS

AT the top of the movement, touch your glute to make sure it's nice and tight.

DO not hyperextend your back.

KEEP your body as straight as you can. Do drop your hips when you bring your knee to your chest.

Strength Training

A1: Reverse Lunge

LOCATION: HOME OR GYM

This exercise targets/strengthens the quadriceps, hamstrings, and glutes of the front leg while elongating the hip flexors and quadriceps of the trailing leg.

Note: Start this exercise with your less-dominant leg.

Sets: 3

Reps: 8 to 10 per side

Load: To be determined

Tempo: 3-0-1-0

Rest interval: Up to 10 seconds

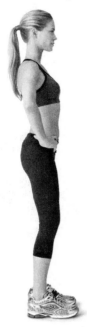

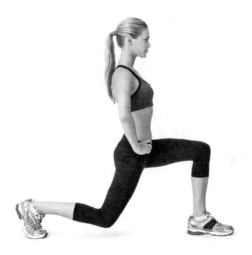

START POSITION

STAND with your feet hip-width apart, spine straight, chest up, shoulders down and back. If you're using dumbbells, hold them down at your sides, your palms facing in.

IF you are not using dumbbells, place your hands on your hips.

THE MOVEMENT

STEP back with your right leg and place your weight on the ball of your foot. At the same time, bend your trailing leg so that your knee almost touches the floor.

PRESS into your left heel as you stand up and return to the start position. Repeat on the same side, then switch sides to complete the set.

TIPS

KEEP your weight on your front heel.

MAINTAIN an upright posture throughout the exercise.

TRY to keep your hips and shoulders square. Do not rotate your hips or shoulders.

IF possible, perform this exercise in front of a mirror so you can more easily maintain good form.

A2: Flat Dumbbell Fly

LOCATION: HOME OR GYM

This exercise predominantly targets the muscles of the chest and anterior deltoids.

Sets: 3

Reps: 8 to 10

Load: To be determined

Tempo: 3-0-1-0

Rest interval: Up to 10 seconds

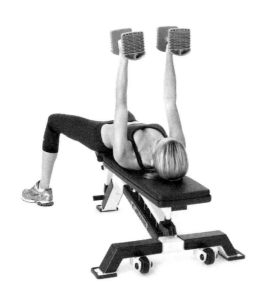
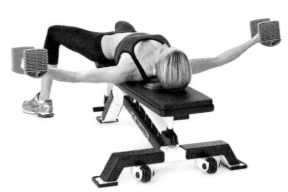

START POSITION

LIE on a flat bench and raise the dumbbells directly over your shoulders, palms facing each other.

THE MOVEMENT

KEEPING a slight bend in your elbows, move your arms out to the side and away from your body.

RETURN to the start position, with the dumbbells directly over your shoulders.

REPEAT to complete the set.

TIPS

RETRACT your shoulder blades slightly, keep your chest up, and arch your lower back slightly.

ON the downward portion of the movement, you should feel a significant stretch in the muscles of your chest.

AS you raise the dumbbells back up, contract your chest muscles.

MAINTAIN a slight bend in your elbows throughout the entire movement.

A3, B3, C3: Skipping Rope

LOCATION: HOME OR GYM

This exercise targets the entire body.

Sets: 3

Reps: 45 to 120 seconds

Load: Body weight

Tempo: Moderate to fast

Rest interval: 60 to 90 seconds

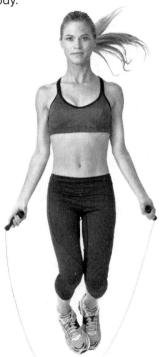

START POSITION

GRIP the handles with your thumb and index finger, with a comfortable but firm grip. Keep your elbows close to your sides.

THE MOVEMENT

MAKE small circles with wrists as you turn the rope.

KEEP your torso relaxed. Look straight ahead.

JUMP only high enough to clear the rope. As you jump, the rope should touch the surface lightly.

TIPS

Buy a good rope. Most sporting-goods stores sell high-quality ropes.

Buy the correct length. Most ropes are at least 9 feet—long enough if you're under 6 feet tall. (If you're taller, purchase a 10-foot rope.) Another good test: Step one foot in the middle of the rope; the handles should reach up to your armpits.

Jump on a shock-absorbent surface. A wood floor is perfect; a gym mat, okay. Never skip rope on concrete.

If you're new to skipping rope, be patient. Skill before conditioning. Think of your rope sessions as skill workouts.

Start with short, frequent sessions. If you're a beginner, 45 to 60 seconds of continuous skipping is plenty. If you're at an intermediate to advanced level of fitness, work up to 2 minutes without stopping.

B1: Single-Leg Romanian Deadlift

LOCATION: HOME OR GYM

This exercise targets the hamstrings and glutes of the weight-bearing leg, the glute of the extended leg, and the core.

Sets: 3	
Reps: 8 to 10 per side	
Load: To be determined	
Tempo: 2-1-1-0	
Rest interval: Up to 10 seconds	

NOTES

BEGIN this exercise with your less-dominant leg.

BEGINNERS: Use a dowel rod for balance, if needed. Hold it like a staff in the hand opposite your weight-bearing leg.

INTERMEDIATE/ADVANCED: If you have the balance and strength, hold two light dumbbells in front of your body.

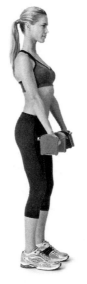
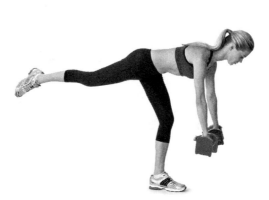

START POSITION

STAND with your feet slightly closer than hip-width apart, arms fully extended with dumbbells in each hand (palms facing thighs).

THE MOVEMENT

SHIFT your weight onto your left leg.

LIFT your other leg off the floor and move it slightly behind you, so all of your weight rests on your left leg, with your knee in a slight bend.

MOVE your torso forward and toward the floor as you extend your trailing leg behind you, ideally raising the back leg until it's parallel to the floor.

SQUEEZE the glute of your left leg as you return to the start position.

REPEAT all reps on one side, then switch sides to complete the set.

TIPS

AT the bottom of the movement, you should feel a stretch in your hamstrings. If you don't, you've placed more load on your lower back, and your knees may be bending too soon.

MAINTAIN good spinal alignment throughout this exercise. Do not round your back.

IF your hamstrings are tight, shorten the range of motion.

B2: Incline Prone Reverse Fly

LOCATION: HOME OR GYM

This exercise predominantly targets the muscles of the upper back (rhomboids and trapezius) and the backs of the shoulder muscles (posterior deltoids).

Sets: 3

Reps: 8 to 10

Load: To be determined

Tempo: 2-0-1-1

Rest interval: Up to 10 seconds

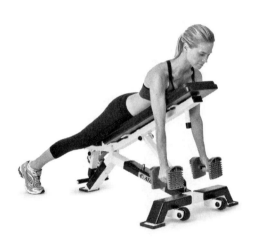 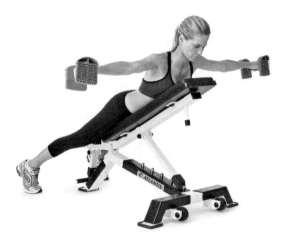

START POSITION

LIE facedown with your chest supported on a 30° incline bench, and hold the dumbbells, palms facing each other and arms straight, directly under the shoulders.

THE MOVEMENT

RAISE your arms directly out to your sides, up to shoulder height, keeping your palms facing the floor.

RETURN to the start position.

REPEAT to complete the set.

TIPS

KEEP your arms in line with your shoulders.

SQUEEZE your shoulder blades together throughout this exercise, especially at the top of the movement.

C1: Standing Dumbbell Curl

LOCATION: HOME OR GYM

This exercise targets the biceps and forearms.

Sets: 3

Reps: 8 to 10

Load: To be determined

Tempo: 3-0-1-0

Rest interval: Up to 10 seconds

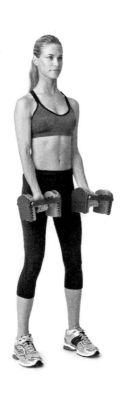
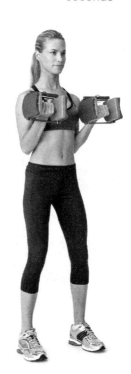

START POSITION

STAND facing a mirror and grasp the dumbbells with your hands facing away from your body. Rest the dumbbells against your thighs.

ADJUST your posture: spine long, chest lifted, shoulders down and back.

THE MOVEMENT

TIGHTEN your biceps and slowly raise the dumbbells. Bring the dumbbells as close to your shoulders as possible.

LOWER and return to the start position.

REPEAT to complete the set.

TIPS

DON'T move your upper arms forward or backward. Only your forearms should move.

KEEP wrists straight and core tight.

C2: Prone Knee Pull-In on Swiss Ball

LOCATION: HOME OR GYM

This exercise targets the core musculature and hip flexors. It also benefits shoulder stability.

Sets: 3

Reps: 8 to 10

Load: Body weight

Tempo: 2-0-2-0

Rest interval: Up to 10 seconds

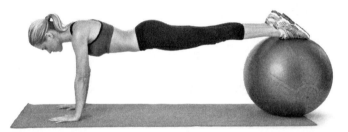
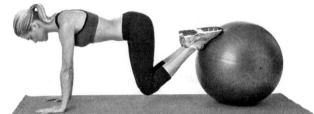

START POSITION

GET in the pushup position with the tops of your feet on the ball. Keep your arms locked and right beneath you. Your body should form a straight line.

THE MOVEMENT

CONTRACT your abdominal muscles slightly. Pull your knees toward your body as far as you can without rounding your lower back.

REVERSE the motion by extending your legs and return to the start position.

REPEAT to complete the set.

TIPS

KEEP your back straight; do not let it sag.

IF you're a beginner, you may start the movement with your shins on the ball.

Energy System Training: Treadmill

If you don't have access to a treadmill, you can walk and run outdoors.

WEEK 1 (25 TO 28 MINUTES TOTAL), EST-9

WARMUP: 5 minutes, 3½ mph, 0 incline; build intensity with each passing minute

WORKOUT: 60 seconds of work (zone 4, RPE 7 to 8), followed by 120 seconds of recovery (zones 1 to 2, RPE 1 to 4); repeat 5 or 6 times

COOLDOWN: 5 minutes, 3½ mph, 0 incline, very low intensity

WEEK 2 (23.5 TO 28 MINUTES TOTAL), EST-10

WARMUP: 5 minutes, 3½ mph, 0 incline; build intensity with each passing minute

WORKOUT: 45 seconds of work (zones 4 to 5, RPE 7 to 10), followed by 90 seconds of recovery (zones 1 to 2, RPE 1 to 4); repeat 6 to 8 times

COOLDOWN: 5 minutes, 3½ mph, 0 incline, very low intensity

WEEK 3 (23½ TO 28 MINUTES TOTAL), EST-11

WARMUP: 5 minutes, 3½ mph, 0 incline; build intensity with each passing minute

WORKOUT: 30 seconds of work (zones 4 to 5, RPE 7 to 10), followed by 60 seconds of recovery (zones 1 to 2, RPE 1 to 4); repeat 8 to 10 times

COOLDOWN: 5 minutes, 3½ mph, 0 incline, very low intensity

WEEK 4 (25½ MINUTES TOTAL), EST-12

WARMUP: 5 minutes, 3½ mph, 0 incline; build intensity with each passing minute

WORKOUT:

A: 30 seconds of work (zone 5, RPE 9 to 10), followed by 60 seconds of recovery (zones 1 to 2, RPE 1 to 4); repeat 3 times

B: 45 seconds of work (zones 4 to 5, RPE 7 to 10), followed by 60 seconds of recovery (zones 1 to 2, RPE 1 to 4); repeat 3 times

C: 60 seconds of work (zone 4, RPE 7 to 8), followed by 60 seconds of recovery (zones 1 to 2, RPE 1 to 4); repeat 3 times

COOLDOWN: 5 minutes, 3½ mph, 0 incline, very low intensity

EST RECOVERY SESSION (TREADMILL, STATIONARY BIKE, OR ELLIPTICAL MACHINE), EST-R

WARMUP: 3 to 5 minutes, TBD; slowly increase speed over the course of the warmup

WORKOUT: 30 to 45 minutes (zone 2, RPE 3 to 4)

COOLDOWN: 3 to 5 minutes, TBD, very low intensity

ENERGY SYSTEM TRAINING POST-WORKOUT

FOAM rolling sequence (pages 42 to 45)

STATIC stretching (pages 45 to 47)

PHASE 3 NUTRITION
Phase 3 at a Glance

> **WEEKS 1 TO 4**
>
> - Address estrogen dominance.
>
> - Reconsider hormonal birth control/HRT.
>
> - Rev up your lean hormones.
>
> - Add Phase 3 supplements.

When a man hits the gym a few extra times a week or gives up ice cream for a few days, he's often rewarded with a six-pack. For most women, those same efforts produce few results.

Why? Two words: sex hormones.

When it comes to fat loss, the impact of estrogen, progesterone, and testosterone is often overlooked. That's surprising, as even a casual glance at men's and women's bodies displays a striking difference in where each sex stores body fat.

In Chapter 5, you learned how estrogen dominance can endanger a woman's health and wreak havoc on her weight. Excess body fat, an unhealthy diet, medications, and an environment rife with endocrine disruptors can cause estrogen dominance. Too much stress adds to the burden as well. Stress raises cortisol and, subsequently, insulin, which can pack on the fat, thus increasing overall estrogen via aromatization (wherein body fat converts testosterone to estrogen).

In Phase 3, you'll continue to follow the eating plan we laid out in Phases 1 and 2 and also take steps to lower your estrogen burden and maximize those lean, mean hormones, testosterone and growth hormone. You stand to lose a significant amount of body fat. Your PMS or perimenopausal symptoms are likely to ease as well, not to mention your complexion will become more clear.

Review the sections on estrogen, progesterone, testosterone, and growth hormone in Chapter 5 if you need to, then follow the suggestions on the next page.

ADDRESS ESTROGEN DOMINANCE

In Phase 3, you will remove as many excess estrogens from your environment as you can. It's not easy—in fact, you probably can't get rid of them all. But this checklist can help.

> Remove as many excess estrogens from your environment as you can.

- **Rid your home of conventional cleaners that can cause damage to your health and the environment.** Use more natural brands such as Mrs. Meyer's Clean Day, Method, and Seventh Generation. See www.sixwise.com for more info on household chemicals.

- **Choose organic produce whenever possible** to avoid estrogenic pesticides.

- **Choose clean, organic, free-range, grass-fed, and hormone-free proteins** as often as possible.

- **Avoid or minimize strong dietary phytoestrogens** (namely, soy), and use herbal phytoestrogens under the guidance of a nutritional medicine practitioner.

- **Minimize alcohol consumption.**

- **Use glass containers for food and drink.** If you use plastic containers to store food, never microwave them. Avoid soft plastic water bottles as much as possible—if you can't use glass, opt for metal bottles, such as SIGG and Klean Kanteen.

- **Switch to paraben- and phthalate-free cosmetics and body- and hair-care products,** such as Jurlique, Weleda, Earth Science, Devita Rx, John Masters Organics, and Aubrey Organics. (Read your labels—even at health-food stores, not all products are chemical free.) Other resources include:

  - www.bodybyhardware.com or www.betterbydrbrooke.com
  - www.lanisimpson.com for paraben-free, natural, doctor-developed skin care
  - www.cosmeticsdatabase.com for safety information on chemicals found in beauty products
  - www.sallyhansennaturalbeauty.com for paraben-free makeup, inspired by Carmindy from TLC's *What Not to Wear*

RECONSIDER HORMONAL BIRTH CONTROL AND CONVENTIONAL HRT

Many women who use a hormonal method of birth control (the Pill, Depo-Provera, or the Mirena IUD) and the synthetic hormone replacement therapy (HRT) prescribed for menopausal symptoms gain weight—and estrogen is likely a factor.

Why did you pack on 10 pounds from the Pill when your best friend swears by hers?

We react differently to hormonal birth control because we all have a unique estrogen/progesterone balance. Also, some women's livers detoxify or "clear" estrogen better than others, so they handle hormonal medications more easily.

If you gained weight with the Pill or had significant side effects (mood swings, water retention, breast swelling, etc.), then you probably do not detoxify estrogen well and will have a difficult time losing weight while on birth-control pills. A non-hormone-secreting IUD or condoms will be a better contraceptive option for you, your physique, and your health.

In addition to use as contraception, birth-control pills are often prescribed to treat high-estrogen/low-progesterone-related issues, such as PMS, painful periods, or acne. But this gives an estrogen-dominant situation more estrogen!

Excess estrogen from these synthetic hormones can worsen estrogen dominance and disrupt thyroid hormone (more on that in Phase 4). Beyond that, the synthetic progestins in Mirena and some birth-control pills seem to increase fat storage in their own right, while conventional HRT and synthetic birth-control hormones increase the burden on the liver because it must clear more estrogen.

If you are in perimenopause or menopause and use HRT, look into bioidentical hormones. Chemically similar to the hormones your body produces, bioidentical hormones seem to cause fewer problems than conventional HRT does.

A salivary hormone test, along with other functional tests, can reveal your current hormonal landscape and how best to support it with nutrition, supplements, and bioidentical hormones, if

most deodorants stink

Among the more problematic personal-care products are deodorants that contain parabens. Most breast cancers occur in the upper outer quadrant of the breast (the area next to the armpit), so rubbing exogenous estrogens into that area is a terrible idea! Natural deodorants that we love include Weleda's spray deodorant in Wild Rose, Sage, and Citrus (available at www.bodybyhardware.com) and Lavanila's The Healthy Deodorant (available at www.sephora.com and www.lavanila.com). However, good ol' baking soda works like a charm! Try this recipe.

- Place ½ to 1 teaspoon of baking soda in your palm.
- Add a small amount of water and mix into a paste.
- Apply to your underarms and let dry.

If you still notice body odor, swab your underarms with rubbing alcohol two or three times per week. The alcohol will kill the bacteria that cause odor.

Important point: Neither baking soda nor the Weleda deodorant is an antiperspirant, so you will continue to sweat. But your body expels toxins and other gunk through sweat. That's why we recommend deodorants over antiperspirants.

If a special occasion or high-stress situation demands dry underarms, use a conventional deodorant/antiperspirant. When the heat is off, so to speak, you can go back to more natural options that reduce your exposure to estrogenic preservatives.

losing weight after 40

Most women know that, after the age of 40, you'll likely find it difficult to shed fat, unless you've maintained a lean, muscular physique throughout your 30s.

One reason: You may have low muscle mass due to low protein intake, low testosterone, not lifting weights, or various lifestyle habits that reduce insulin sensitivity. Another reason: As women age, they experience an overt or relative deficiency in progesterone and lower levels of testosterone, which creates at least a relative estrogen dominance. (If they are overweight or already have an overt estrogen dominance, this effect is amplified.) In other words, as you age you become more estrogen dominant, even though you are producing less estrogen.

When you enter perimenopause or menopause, ovarian production of your sex hormones dwindles. Soon only your adrenal glands will produce progesterone and testosterone, and not much at that. If you battled constant stress in your younger years (and what woman hasn't?), then it will be even harder for your adrenals to produce these sex hormones. It becomes more important than ever to manage stress, eat regularly, get adequate sleep, train intensely (particularly by doing strength training and avoiding long-duration, moderate-intensity cardio), and consume a diet high in vegetables, fiber, and protein and lower in starchy carbs.

warranted. To find out whether bioidentical hormones are right for you, seek out a licensed naturopathic doctor or functional medicine doctor. (You can find licensed practitioners in your area at www.naturopathic.org or www.functional medicine.org.) If you're currently on conventional HRT, don't stop on your own—speak with your doctor first.

Get a minimum of 7 to 8 hours of restful sleep per night. To enhance the secretion of growth hormone while you sleep, eat your last bite of food 2 to 3 hours before bedtime.

REV UP YOUR LEAN HORMONES

The tips below will help you optimize your body's release of both testosterone and growth hormone.

- **Sleep deep and on an empty stomach.** Get a minimum of 7 to 8 hours of restful sleep per night. To enhance the secretion of growth hormone while you sleep, eat your last bite of food 2 to 3 hours before bedtime.

- **Stick to the 3-to-4-hour rule.** If you eat more frequently than this, you will hinder the release of growth hormone.

- **Skip sugars and "sugar water" with exercise.** Before and during a workout, avoid high-carbohydrate foods or drinks, particularly those that contain fructose or high-fructose corn syrup. In the presence of sugar, cortisol will not rise during your workouts. Along with lactic acid, cortisol signals your body to release glucagon, testosterone, and growth hormone. This combo will help you burn fat for hours and even days after your workouts.

- **Avoid high-fat meals post-workout.** Excess fatty acids will blunt the growth-hormone response of those intense workouts. So don't add nuts, nut butter, coconut oil, or coconut milk to your Recovery Shake.

- **Add a few low-intensity walks to your workout program.** If you have a lot of weight to lose, you may want to add some long, easy walks—ideally, first thing in the morning, before breakfast—to the EST workouts. Recharge, get fresh air, catch up with a friend, or listen to an audiobook—this exercise is not meant to be intense. Don't add long-duration, moderate-intensity cardio like jogging, however. It will lower your precious amounts of testosterone and worsen estrogen dominance.

- **Burn, baby, burn.** Follow this guideline when you lift weights: Once you can complete 3 sets of 10 reps, raise your weights 2½ to 5 pounds (upper body) and 5 to 10 pounds (lower body). Also, push hard enough during your EST sessions to get a good burn in your muscles. The burn is from acidic hydrogen ions. To buffer these, your body forms lactic acid, which serves as fuel for the muscle and triggers the release of glucagon, testosterone, and growth hormone.

> Push hard enough during your EST sessions to get a good burn in your muscles.

- **Fill up on protein.** There are various ways to calculate protein needs based on lean body mass. But who needs a complicated formula? Simply consume 4 to 6 ounces of lean protein at meals and 2 to 4 ounces as a snack.

- **Get frisky.** Regular sexual activity—with or without a partner—boosts testosterone, especially in women.

- **Don't skimp on fat.** Eat adequate healthy fats such as nuts, olives and olive oil, coconut oil, and organic butter.

- **Curtail the cocktails.** Limit alcohol or avoid it completely. Extra booze calories can pack on pounds. Worse, alcohol enhances the aromatization of testosterone

your sex hormone cheat sheet

HORMONE IMBALANCE	LIFESTYLE TRIGGERS	BODY-FAT SITES
Estrogen dominance	Environmental estrogens in food, cosmetics, plastics, cleaning products, etc.; birth control; conventional HRT; alcohol	Hips, thighs (particularly hamstring area), breasts; secondarily, testosterone sites (triceps and chest)
Low progesterone	High stress or anything that elevates estrogen	Secondarily, estrogen sites and waist (in conjunction with cortisol and testosterone)
Low testosterone	High estrogen and high stress; lack of sleep; long-duration cardiovascular exercise; lack of intense weight training; inadequate protein intake or a low-fat diet; alcohol	Triceps and chest; secondarily, hips, thighs, butt, and breasts, as well as waist
Low growth hormone	Lack of sleep; alcohol; eating too frequently or too close to bedtime; eating high-sugar foods before/during exercise or a high-fat meal after exercise	Medial calf (lower leg); above the front of the knee

to estrogen. And if you drink to the point of intoxication, you can lower your testosterone levels for several days.

ADD PHASE 3 SUPPLEMENTS

Diet, exercise, and lifestyle are the champs of balancing sex hormones. That said, several nutrients can help you shift the balance in favor of leanness.

TO MANAGE ESTROGEN

Herbs

Take daily as directed on the label or in the doses below.

To modulate estrogen balance:

- Grapeseed extract, 200 milligrams standardized proanthocyanidins, 1 to 3 times daily

- Resveratrol, 400 milligrams, 1 to 3 times daily
- Curcumin, 800 milligrams, 1 to 3 times daily

To *inhibit aromatization of testosterone to estrogen:*

- Chrysin is poorly absorbed from the gut, so use a topical formulation (found at www.bodybyhardware.com).

    Note: Vitex (chasteberry), dong quai, and black cohosh (*Cimicifuga racemosa*) are phytoestrogenic herbs. Use them only under a doctor's care to ensure they are right for your particular hormonal imbalances.

Nutrients

- DIM (diindolylmethane) is a derivative of indole-3-carbinol and helps your liver detoxify estrogen. DIM is difficult to absorb, so look for formulas that are emulsified and have nutrients (such as lecithin) that enhance absorption. Taking 100 to 600 milligrams per day can help lower estrogen burden; however, we recommend you seek the advice of a health-care practitioner to determine the best dose for you.

- B_6 is vital to liver detoxification of estrogens and other hormones. You should know that some people experience numbness and other neurological symptoms when they take doses over 200 milligrams per day. Before you add a B_6 supplement, add up the amount contained in all of your supplements to avoid going over without supervision.

- Zinc is an aromatase inhibitor; take a minimum of 30 milligrams per day. While important to estrogen/testosterone balance, this nutrient can, if taken in excess, create other nutrient deficiencies. Test your zinc "status" with zinc tally liquids (available from a nutritional medicine practitioner or at www.bodybyhardware.com; follow the directions on the bottle) and supplement in 30-milligram increments for mild, moderate, or severe deficiencies.

Foods

Fruits and vegetables are great aromatase inhibitors and estrogen modulators—particularly raw or steamed cruciferous veggies such as broccoli, Brussels sprouts, cabbage, radish, rutabaga, kohlrabi, turnips, collard greens, kale, arugula, and watercress, as they contain indoles and isothiocyanates and modulate and detoxify estrogens. (Don't microwave or boil them; these cooking methods destroy many of the active compounds.)

Fresh ground flaxseed (not preground) is also an aromatase inhibitor. See page 81 for how to use fresh ground flaxseed.

TO BOOST TESTOSTERONE

Herbs

Take daily as directed on the label or in the doses below.

- Tribulus, 200 milligrams
- Maca root, 200 milligrams
- Ashwagandha, 200 milligrams

Nutrients

- L-carnitine increases testosterone receptor number and sensitivity. Often, high doses are necessary for results, and a pure L form of carnitine is a must. Consider Ultimate Liquid Carnitine (Hardware), 1 to 2 teaspoons 1 to 3 times daily.

  Note: Carnitine can be stimulating, so be sure to take all doses before 5 p.m. Also, long-term supplementation with high doses of L-carnitine can hinder thyroid function. For long-term use of this nutrient, seek the advice of a nutritional medicine practitioner.

- Find a multivitamin that contains at least 200 micrograms of selenium or take it in an individual supplement.

- Libido Stim-F (Designs for Health), 1 or 2 capsules with meals 3 times per day

- Ultimate Zinc (Hardware), 1 to 3 capsules daily with food

Foods

To stimulate growth hormone, eat lean, high-quality proteins and be diligent with your Recovery Shake recipe.

CHAPTER 11

Phase 4: Ultimate You

WELCOME TO PHASE 4! By now, you should look—and feel—quite different than when you began the program. You've likely lost inches, pounds, and body fat and gained lean muscle and a new outlook on life.

Prepare yourself—this last phase will challenge you. In this phase's strength-training sessions, you will perform full-body resistance circuits with minimal rest between exercises, which will turn up the caloric expenditure. The EST workouts will take your conditioning to another level—and by changing apparatuses, you'll get the added benefit of increased physical and mental stimulation.

In Phase 4, your goals are to continue to increase lean muscle mass, decrease body fat, and raise the intensity and challenge of the anaerobic interval training. You'll train 6 times a week—3 strength-training sessions, 2 EST sessions, and 1 EST recovery session.

If you've been training at home, you must join a gym for this phase, as the strength-training exercises and EST workouts require more diversified equipment.

ULTIMATE YOU WORKOUT

- **STRENGTH TRAINING:** You will perform 3 different programs—A, B, and C. All 3 are total-body circuits. In other words, you will perform 1 set of each exercise, with minimum rest, then move to the next exercise. When you complete all exercises in the sequence, you will rest for the prescribed amount of time, then repeat the circuit 2 or 3 more times.

  Keep in mind that every gym is set up or laid out differently. Look closely at the exercises in Phase 4 and at what equipment you will need. Next, look closely at your gym and see where you can set up your circuit. You will need to set up your circuit so that you have all the required weights and equipment close at hand in order to stick to the short rest periods between exercises.

And keep in mind that you may be the only woman on the squat rack or doing a barbell bench press—so get used to sharing that equipment with the boys. No need to be intimidated; in fact, you might even gain more respect from the guys.

- EST: In this phase, you'll push your anaerobic interval training to another level by varying the apparatuses. You'll do from 15 to 31 minutes, including warmup and cooldown, on a combination of a stationary bike along with a rower and/or VersaClimber. Don't forget to use your unique heart-rate and RPE training zones. These workouts will intensify each week, which will ultimately help you get leaner.

  You'll also perform a weekly EST recovery workout—36 to 55 minutes (including warmup and cooldown) of low-intensity steady-state cardio, using the treadmill, bike, or elliptical.

- RECOVERY: Always foam roll after each workout in both your EST and resistance-training sessions. Perform static stretching after each EST session, and feel free to do it after resistance-training sessions, too (after you've foam rolled). You can also perform foam rolling before the dynamic warmup of the resistance-training session, particularly if you're feeling sore or tight. And feel free to incorporate some other recovery techniques from Chapter 4 as well. Remember: Muscles repair, rebuild, and strengthen when you rest, not when you train.

ULTIMATE YOU NUTRITION

If you're at or near your goal, congratulations! If you're still struggling or have hit a plateau, we've got a few tricks up our sleeves that can get your program back on track. In Phase 4, you will:

- **Tweak/troubleshoot thyroid hormone and neurotransmitters (brain chemicals).** If the fat isn't coming off quickly enough, tinkering with them can help.

- **Turn up your metabolic furnace.** If your thyroid is running on low, you'll stoke it with a unique, healthy fat; protect it from environmental damage; and give it the nutrients it needs to function better.

- **Get to know your neurotransmitters.** You'll learn how these brain chemicals may be feeding your cravings—and derailing your program—and what to eat to regulate your moods.

- **Try "carb patterning" and "carb cycling."** If your fat loss has stalled, these techniques can help. Carb patterning keeps your brain chemicals at the right levels at the right times of day, while carb cycling can help spark a sluggish metabolism, break a plateau, and boost feel-good brain chemicals.

PHASE 4 WORKOUT AT A GLANCE

We've designed 3 separate strength-training routines for this phase: Programs A, B, and C. For the next 4 weeks, you will alternate between them.

The EST sessions will be different each week, except for the recovery session, which is the same as Phases 1 through 3.

- HOW LONG: 4 weeks

- HOW OFTEN: 6 times a week

  - 3 Phase 4 strength-training sessions

  - 2 EST interval sessions

  - 1 EST recovery session

- GOALS: To continue to increase lean muscle mass; continue to decrease body fat; raise the intensity/challenge of EST

WEEK	MONDAY	TUESDAY	WEDNESDAY	THURSDAY	FRIDAY	SATURDAY	SUNDAY
1	Strength 4-A	EST-13	Strength 4-B	EST-13	Strength 4-C	EST-R	Off
2	Strength 4-A	EST-14	Strength 4-B	EST-14	Strength 4-C	EST-R	Off
3	Strength 4-A	EST-15	Strength 4-B	EST-15	Strength 4-C	EST-R	Off
4	Strength 4-A	EST-16	Strength 4-B	EST-16	Strength 4-C	EST-R	Off

PHASE 4 STRENGTH-TRAINING PROGRAM A

Dynamic Warmup

	Sets	Reps	Load	Tempo	Rest	Intensity
A: Forward Lunge with Elbow to Instep/ Straight-Leg Extension	1	5/side	b/w	Slow	—	Low
B: Drop-Step Crossover Squat	1	5/side	b/w	Slow	30 sec	Low

Activation Drills

	Sets	Reps	Load	Tempo	Rest	Intensity
A: Mini-Band Walking— Diagonal	1	10/side	TBD	Slow	—	Low
B: Bird Dog	1	5/side	b/w	Slow	30 sec	Low

Strength Training

	Sets	Reps	Load	Tempo	Rest
A1: Clean-Grip Deadlift	3–4	10–12	TBD	3-0-1-0	Up to 15 sec
A2: Flat Barbell Bench Press*	3–4	10–12	TBD	3-0-1-0	Up to 15 sec
A3: Bulgarian Dumbbell Split Squat	3–4	10–12/ side	TBD	3-0-1-0	Up to 15 sec
A4: Close-Grip Chinup	3–4	10–12	TBD	3-0-1-0	Up to 15 sec
A5: Dumbbell Lateral Raise	3–4	10–12	b/w	3-0-1-0	Up to 15 sec
A6: Half-Kneeling Cable Chop	3–4	10–12/ side	TBD	2-0-2-0	Up to 120 sec

*Or substitute with Flat Dumbbell Bench Press

Dynamic Warmup

A: Forward Lunge with Elbow to Instep/Straight-Leg Extension

LOCATION: GYM

This exercise elongates the hip flexor of the back leg and the glute and the hamstrings of the front leg.

Sets: 1
Reps: 5 per side
Load: Body weight
Tempo: Slow
Rest interval: —
Intensity: Low

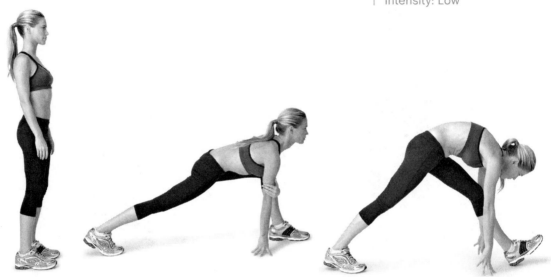

START POSITION

STAND with your arms at your sides and your feet together.

THE MOVEMENT

STEP forward into a lunge with your left foot.

PLACE your right hand on the floor and your left elbow to the inside of your left shin, and hold the stretch for 1 to 2 seconds.

PLACE your left hand outside of your foot and lift your left toes toward your shin as you push your hips toward the ceiling (feeling the stretch in your left hamstring).

DROP your hips and step into the next repetition with your right leg.

CONTINUE until you have completed 5 lunges on each side.

TIPS

DO not let your back knee touch the floor.

SQUEEZE your back glute during the stretch.

B: Drop-Step Crossover Squat

LOCATION: GYM

This exercise helps elongate the outer glute area of the front leg.

Sets: 1
Reps: 5 per side
Load: Body weight
Tempo: Slow
Rest interval: 30 seconds
Intensity: Low

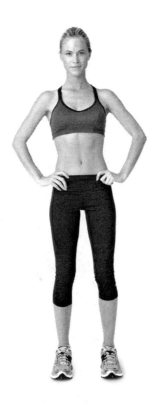

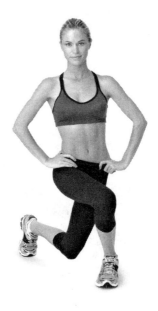

START POSITION

STAND with your feet together and your hands on your hips. Keep your shoulders square and level.

THE MOVEMENT

BRING your left foot back and around behind your body, as if to perform a curtsy.

WITH your left foot behind you, bend both knees and begin to lower your hips down and back, until your left knee is almost touching the floor.

KEEP your torso upright and shoulder blades slightly drawn together throughout the movement.

PRESS back up and return to the start position. Perform the same movement, but bring your right foot behind you and alternate until you've completed 5 reps on each side.

TIPS

DO not let your back knee touch the floor.

KEEP your shoulders and hips level and facing forward.

Activation Drills

A: Mini-Band Walking—Diagonal

LOCATION: GYM

This exercise targets the glutes.

Sets: 1
Reps: 10 per side
Load: To be determined
Tempo: Slow
Rest interval: —
Intensity: Low

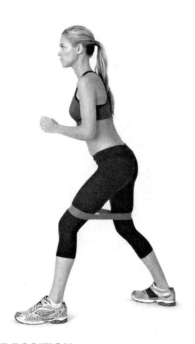 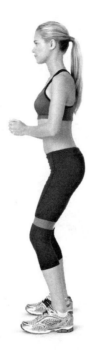 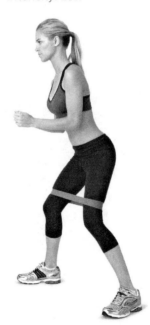

START POSITION

WRAP your miniband around both legs just above your knees.

THE MOVEMENT

TAKE a diagonal step back with your right foot. Your front knee is still bent in the same position and your back leg is extended with the knee slightly bent.

BRING your front foot back and in to return to the start position.

TAKE a diagonal step back with your left foot. Continue to alternate until you've completed 5 reps on each side.

TIP

KEEP your hips and shoulders facing forward throughout the exercise.

B: Bird Dog

LOCATION: GYM

This exercise activates the glutes and develops the stabilizing muscles in the back.

Sets: 1
Reps: 5 per side
Load: Body weight
Tempo: Slow
Rest interval: 30 seconds
Intensity: Low

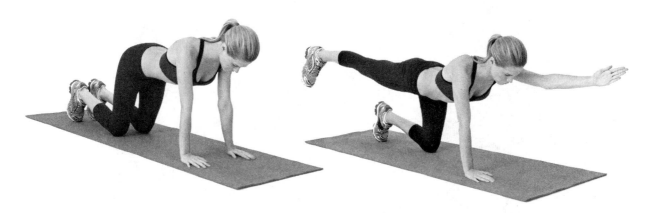

START POSITION

START on your hands and knees; align your knees under your hips and your palms under your shoulders. Look at the floor and tuck your chin to your neck.

SLIGHTLY contract your core muscles.

THE MOVEMENT

SQUEEZING your right glute, extend your right leg straight behind you, in line with your torso, as you simultaneously extend your left arm straight out.

HOLD for 1 to 2 seconds.

RETURN to the start position, but do not let your knee touch the ground.

REPEAT all reps on one side, then switch to perform reps on the other side to complete the set.

TIPS

WHEN returning to the start position, let your knee hover just above the floor.

CONTRACT your working glute and your core muscles throughout the exercise.

Strength Training

A1: Clean-Grip Deadlift

LOCATION: GYM

This exercise targets the glutes, quads, hamstrings, lower back, and core.

Sets: 3 or 4

Reps: 10 to 12

Load: To be determined

Tempo: 3-0-1-0

Rest interval: Up to 15 seconds

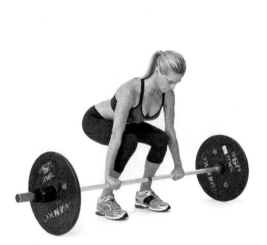 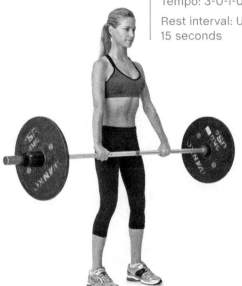

START POSITION

PLACE a loaded bar on the floor and make sure that your shins are touching it.

WITH your feet hip-width apart, bend at your knees and hips and grab the bar with an overhand grip, keeping your hands shoulder-width apart.

LIFT your chest and shift your body weight slightly onto your heels.

THE MOVEMENT

PUSHING down through your heels, contract your glutes and core muscles as you lift the barbell to hip level.

REVERSE the movement by lowering the bar to the tops of your knees, keeping it as close to your body as possible.

TIP

KEEP your shoulder blades down and back throughout the movement.

A2: Flat Barbell Bench Press*

*Or substitute with Flat Dumbbell Bench Press on page 147

LOCATION: GYM

This exercise targets primarily the chest, shoulders, and triceps.

Sets: 3 or 4

Reps: 10 to 12

Load: To be determined

Tempo: 3-0-1-0

Rest interval: Up to 15 seconds

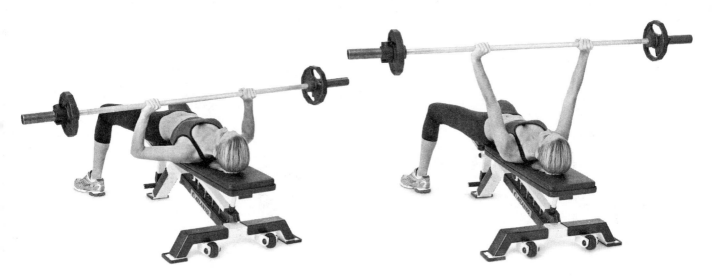

START POSITION

LIE on your back on a flat bench, with your feet planted firmly on either side of the bench (not in front of the bench).

POSITION your body so that your eyes are directly beneath the bar.

DRAW your shoulder blades down and back.

THE MOVEMENT

GRASP the bar in an overhand grip with your hands slightly wider than shoulder-width apart. Carefully unrack the bar and move it out so it is directly above your sternum and your arms are completely straight.

LOWER the bar, keeping your arms at a 45° angle to your torso. As you lower, make sure to tuck your elbows in and keep your shoulders down and back. The bar should move straight down, just touching your chest.

PRESS the bar back up.

REPEAT to complete the set.

TIP

KEEP your elbows in as you raise and lower the bar; do not allow them to flare out.

A3: Bulgarian Dumbbell Split Squat

LOCATION: GYM

This exercise targets the glutes, hamstrings, and quads, as well as the stabilizing muscles of the core.

Sets: 3 or 4

Reps: 10 to 12 per side

Load: To be determined

Tempo: 3-0-1-0

Rest interval: Up to 15 seconds

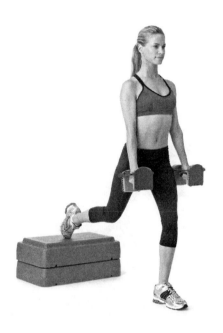
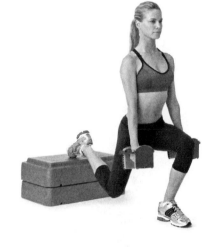

START POSITION

PLACE a 12-inch-high bench or box about 3 feet behind you. Stand with your back to the bench or box with your arms at your sides and a dumbbell in each hand. Keep your head up, your neck straight, and maintain proper spinal alignment.

PLACE your left foot well out in front of the bench or step, and reach backward with your right leg and place the top of that foot on top of the bench or box.

CONTRACT your core muscles.

THE MOVEMENT

KEEPING your chest high and your spine in proper alignment, bend your front knee and lower your body as deeply as possible. Keep the heel of your front foot firmly on the floor.

RETURN to the start position by driving upward.

REPEAT to complete the set, then switch legs.

TIPS

AT the bottom of the movement, the knee of your trailing leg should be just above the floor.

KEEP your torso up and your shoulders down and back throughout the exercise.

YOU should feel a good stretch in the front of your hip and thigh of your trailing leg.

A4: Close-Grip Chinup

LOCATION: GYM

This exercise targets the lats and biceps, as well as the stabilizing muscles of the core.

Sets: 3 or 4

Reps: 10 to 12

Load: To be determined.

Tempo: 3-0-1-0

Rest interval: Up to 15 seconds

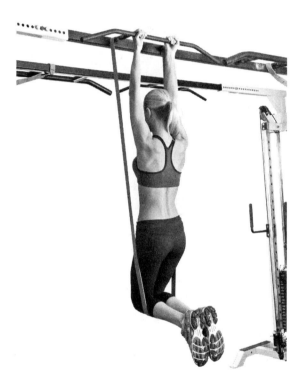 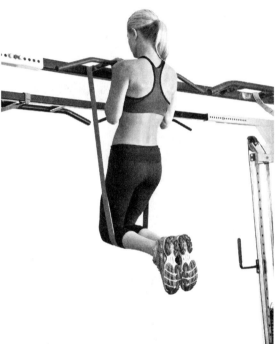

START POSITION

PLACE your hands about 6 inches apart on a chinup bar, with your palms facing you. Let your body hang down and bend your knees slightly.

THE MOVEMENT

PULL your body upward until your chin clears the bar. Make sure you squeeze your shoulder blades together.

RETURN to the start position.

REPEAT to complete the set.

TIP

IF this exercise is too challenging, use a chinup assist machine or a band (as pictured) to help you.

A5: Dumbbell Lateral Raise

LOCATION: GYM

This exercise targets the shoulders.

Note: If you have lower back, neck, or elbow problems, be careful when you perform this exercise.

Sets: 3 or 4

Reps: 10 to 12

Load: To be determined

Tempo: 3-0-1-0

Rest interval: Up to 15 seconds

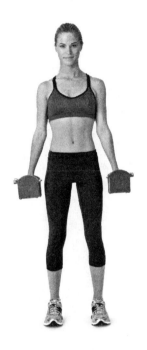 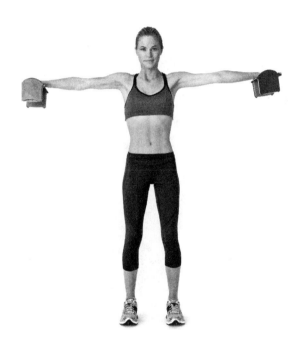

START POSITION

HOLD the dumbbells at your sides, palms facing in. Bend slightly at your hips and knees.

THE MOVEMENT

RAISE your upper arms to your sides until your elbows are at shoulder height. Make sure to keep the height of your elbows above or equal to the height of your wrists.

RETURN to the start position. Repeat to complete the set.

TIPS

DO not let your wrists go above your elbows as you raise the weight. This will target the front of your shoulders, rather than the side of your shoulders.

TO keep your elbows in the correct position as you raise up, tilt the dumbbells down as if you were pouring a jug of water.

BE sure to keep your core braced and engaged.

A6: Half-Kneeling Cable Chop

LOCATION: GYM

This exercise targets the rotator muscles in the torso, particularly the obliques.

Sets: 3 or 4

Reps: 10 to 12 per side

Load: To be determined

Tempo: 2-0-2-0

Rest interval: Up to 120 seconds

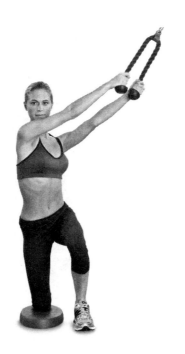 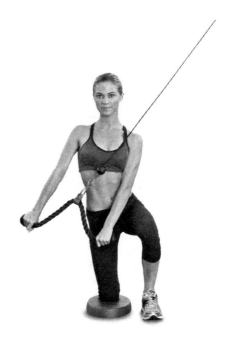

START POSITION

ATTACH a rope handle to the high-cable pulley. Kneel on a pad about 3 feet from the cable machine. Grasp the handle with both hands (as pictured) with body positioned perpendicular to cable machine.

KNEEL on your outside leg, with your inside leg up and your knee bent.

THE MOVEMENT

PULL the handle down toward your chest and continue to press the handle down and across your body.

KEEP hips facing forward and try not to let your torso rotate too much from the lower back, keeping movement in mid and upper spine.

REVERSE the movement and repeat all reps on one side, then switch sides to complete the set.

TIP

AT the finish position, make sure your chest is raised, your shoulders are down and back, and your abdominal muscles are tight.

PHASE 4 STRENGTH-TRAINING PROGRAM B

Dynamic Warmup

	Sets	Reps	Load	Tempo	Rest	Intensity
A: Forward Lunge with Elbow to Instep/ Straight-Leg Extension	1	5/side	b/w	Slow	—	Low
B: Drop-Step Crossover Squat	1	5/side	b/w	Slow	30 sec	Low

Activation Drills

	Sets	Reps	Load	Tempo	Rest	Intensity
A: Mini-Band Walking— Diagonal	1	10/side	TBD	Slow	—	Low
B: Bird Dog	1	5/side	b/w	Slow	30 sec	Low

Strength Training

	Sets	Reps	Load	Tempo	Rest
A1: Back Squat	3–4	10–12	TBD	3-0-1-0	Up to 15 sec
A2: Incline Barbell Bench Press*	3–4	10–12	TBD	3-0-1-0	Up to 15 sec
A3: Dumbbell Stepup	3–4	10–12/ side	TBD	2-0-1-0	Up to 15 sec
A4: Bent-Over Barbell Row**	3–4	10–12	TBD	3-0-1-0	Up to 15 sec
A5: Standing Dumbbell Zottman Curl	3–4	10–12	TBD	3-0-1-0	Up to 15 sec
A6: Half-Kneeling Cable Lift	3–4	10–12/ side	TBD	2-0-2-0	up to 120 sec

*Or substitute with Incline Dumbbell Bench Press

**Or substitute with Single-Arm Dumbbell Row

Dynamic Warmup and Activation Drills

PERFORM the warmups and drills in Program A.

Strength Training

A1: Back Squat

LOCATION: GYM
This exercise primarily targets the quads, hamstrings, glutes, and core.

Sets: 3 or 4

Reps: 10 to 12

Load: To be determined

Tempo: 3-0-1-0

Rest interval: Up to 15 seconds

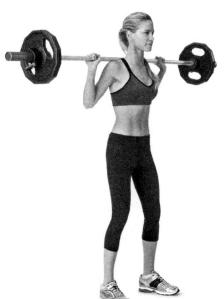

START POSITION

PLACE the bar across your upper back using an overhand grip.

STAND tall and place your spine in proper alignment. Tip your hips slightly back and contract your core muscles hard.

DRAW your shoulder blades together and bring elbows forward.

UNRACK the bar carefully and take a step backward. Position feet shoulder-width apart.

THE MOVEMENT

KEEP lower back arched, bend knees and hips, and descend as deep as you can. Initiate this movement by pushing your hips back. Ideally, at the bottom of the movement, your thighs will be parallel to the floor or slightly lower.

DRIVE upward and return to the start position.

REPEAT to complete the set.

TIPS

KEEP chest up, shoulder blades together, and eyes looking straight ahead.

KEEP core muscles tight and engaged throughout the movement.

A2: Incline Barbell Bench Press*

*Or substitue with Incline Dumbbell Bench Press on page 158

LOCATION: GYM

This exercise targets primarily the upper chest, shoulders, and triceps.

Sets: 3 or 4

Reps: 10 to 12

Load: To be determined

Tempo: 3-0-1-0

Rest interval: Up to 15 seconds

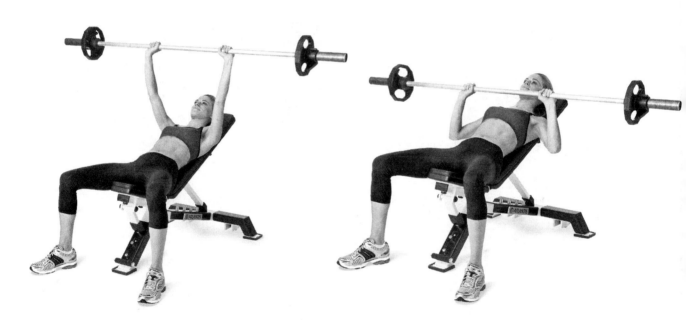

START POSITION

LIE on your back on an incline bench set at 30°.

PLACE your hands about shoulder-width apart, using an overhand grip. Carefully unrack the bar and move it out so it is directly above your sternum, and your arms are completely straight.

THE MOVEMENT

LOWER the bar straight down to your upper chest.

KEEP arms at a 45° angle to your torso. Return to the start position and repeat for 10 to 12 reps.

TIPS

KEEP wrists straight throughout entire movement.

KEEP core tight.

A3: Dumbbell Stepup

LOCATION: GYM

This exercise targets the quads, hamstrings, and glutes.

Sets: 3 or 4

Reps: 10 to 12 per side

Load: To be determined

Tempo: 2-0-1-0

Rest interval: Up to 15 seconds

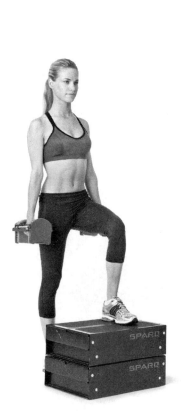
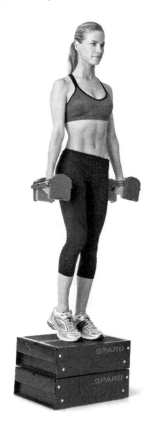

START POSITION

HOLD a pair of dumbbells in your hands at arm's length with palms facing in.

STAND facing a bench or step and place your left foot on it. (Be sure the step or bench is high enough that your left thigh is parallel to the floor.)

THE MOVEMENT

PRESS down through your left heel, raising yourself up until your left leg is fully extended. Your right foot should gently touch the top of the step.

LOWER yourself back down until your right foot touches the floor, keeping your left foot on top of the bench or step.

REPEAT for 10 to 12 reps on your left leg, then switch legs to complete the set.

TIPS

DRAW shoulder blades together, keeping your chest up throughout the movement.

KEEP core tight and engaged at all times.

DON'T push off with foot on floor as you raise yourself up.

A4: Bent-Over Barbell Row*

*Or Single-Arm Dumbbell Row on page 190

LOCATION: GYM

This exercise targets primarily the lats, middle back, and biceps.

Sets: 3 or 4	
Reps: 10 to 12	
Load: To be determined	
Tempo: 3-0-1-0	
Rest interval: Up to 15 seconds	

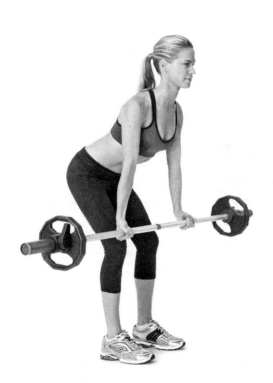
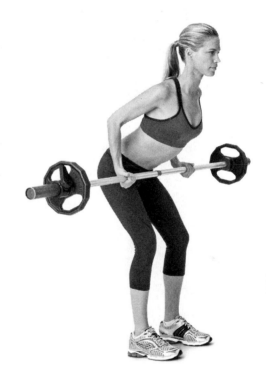

START POSITION

GRAB barbell with underhand grip, hands about shoulder-width apart at arm's length.

BEND at your hips and knees, until torso is about 30° above parallel to the floor.

THE MOVEMENT

PULL the bar up to your abs, slightly above your belly button. Squeeze your shoulder blades together.

RETURN to the start position. Repeat to complete the set.

TIPS

DON'T change the angle of your torso during movement.

KEEP back straight and core engaged throughout entire set.

A5: Standing Dumbbell Zottman Curl

LOCATION: GYM

This exercise targets the biceps and forearms.

Sets: 3 or 4

Reps: 10 to 12

Load: To be determined

Tempo: 3-0-1-0

Rest interval: Up to 15 seconds

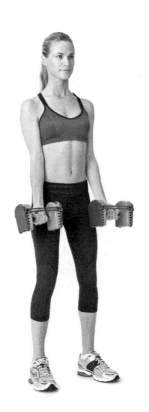
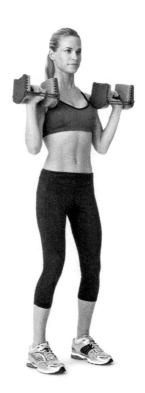

START POSITION

HOLD a pair of dumbbells at arm's length, palms facing away from you with your feet about hip-width apart and knees slightly bent.

THE MOVEMENT

CURL the dumbbells up toward your shoulders without letting your upper arms swing forward or backward.

ROTATE wrists at the top of the movement so that your palms face away from you.

LOWER dumbbells to your sides, arms fully extended (palms facing your thighs).

ROTATE your wrists to the original start position, so that your palms face up. Repeat to complete the set.

TIP

KEEP your core tight.

A6: Half-Kneeling Cable Lift

LOCATION: GYM

This exercise targets the rotator muscles of your torso, particularly the obliques.

Sets: 3 or 4

Reps: 10 to 12 per side

Load: To be determined

Tempo: 2-0-2-0

Rest interval: Up to 120 seconds

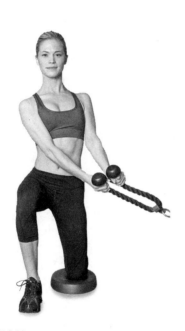 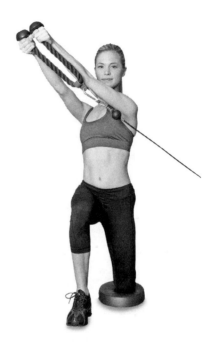

START POSITION

ATTACH a rope handle to the low-cable pulley. Kneel on a pad about 3 feet away from cable machine, grasping the handle with both hands, your body perpendicular to the machine.

KNEEL on your inside leg; bend your outside leg at the knee.

THE MOVEMENT

PULL the handle up toward your chest and continue to pull it up and across your body.

KEEP hips facing forward and try not to let your torso rotate too much from the lower back, keeping movement in mid and upper spine.

REVERSE the movement and repeat all reps on one side, then switch sides to complete the set.

TIP

AT the finish position, make sure your chest is raised, your shoulders are down and back, and your abdominal muscles are tight.

PHASE 4 STRENGTH-TRAINING PROGRAM C

Dynamic Warmup

	Sets	Reps	Load	Tempo	Rest	Intensity
A: Forward Lunge with Elbow to Instep/ Straight-Leg Extension	1	5/side	b/w	Slow	—	Low
B: Drop-Step Crossover Squat	1	5/side	b/w	Slow	30 sec	Low

Activation Drills

	Sets	Reps	Load	Tempo	Rest	Intensity
A: Mini-Band Walking— Diagonal	1	10/side	TBD	Slow	—	Low
B: Bird Dog	1	5/side	b/w	Slow	30 sec	Low

Strength Training

	Sets	Reps	Load	Tempo	Rest
A1: Walking Dumbbell Lunge	3–4	10–12/ side	TBD	3-0-1-0	Up to 15 sec
A2: T-Pushup	3–4	Up to 12/ side	b/w	2-0-2-0	Up to 15 sec
A3: Good Morning	3–4	10–12	TBD	3-0-1-0	Up to 15 sec
A4: Standing Split-Stance High-Pulley Face Pull	3–4	10–12	TBD	3-0-1-0	Up to 15 sec
A5: Dip	3–4	10–12	b/w	3-0-1-0	Up to 15 sec
A6: Hanging Knee Raise	3–4	10–12	b/w	2-0-2-0	Up to 120 sec

Dynamic Warmup and Activation Drills

PERFORM the warmups and drills in Program A.

Strength Training

A1: Walking Dumbbell Lunge

LOCATION: GYM

This exercise targets the quads, glutes, hamstrings, and core.

Sets: 3 or 4

Reps: 10 to 12 per side

Load: To be determined

Tempo: 3-0-1-0

Rest interval: Up to 15 seconds

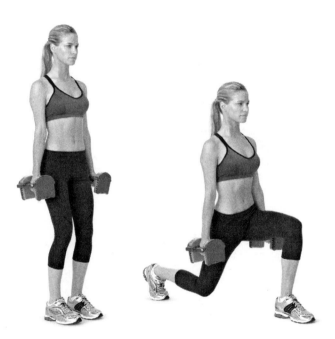
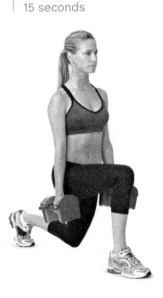

START POSITION:

GRAB a pair of dumbbells and hold them at your sides with palms facing each other.

BEFORE you begin the movement, make sure you think about keeping a tall spine; your shoulder blades should be slightly drawn together, your chest up, and your midsection braced.

THE MOVEMENT:

TAKE a step forward with your left leg and then slowly lower your body until your left knee is bent at least 90°.

PRESS forcefully through your left foot and raise up while bringing your right leg forward so that you are taking a step forward with your right foot now out in front.

CONTINUE to alternate the leg you step forward with until you've completed 10 to 12 reps on each side.

A2: T-Pushup

LOCATION: HOME OR GYM

This exercise targets the muscles of the chest, shoulders, triceps, and core.

Note: If this exercise is too challenging, perform from your knees instead of toes.

Sets: 3 or 4

Reps: Up to 12 per side

Load: Body weight

Tempo: 2-0-2-0

Rest interval: Up to 15 seconds

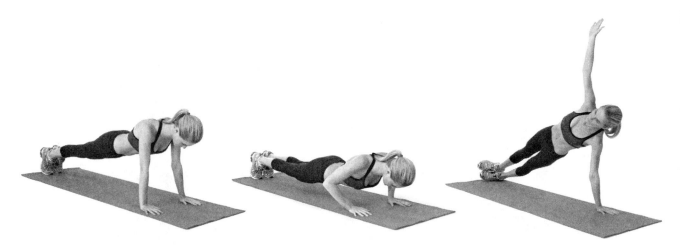

START POSITION

ASSUME a pushup position, feet about hip-width apart, your hands slightly more than shoulder-width apart, with your palms flat on the floor.

THE MOVEMENT

LOWER your body to the floor.

AS you drive back up, rotate to the right side and raise your right arm toward the ceiling so that shoulders and hips are stacked (like a side plank) and arms form a T with your body.

REVERSE movement and repeat on your left side. Continue to alternate sides until you've completed as many as you can, up to 12 per side.

REPEAT, alternating arms, to complete the set.

TIP

DON'T let your hips drop down.

A3: Good Morning

LOCATION: GYM

This exercise targets the glutes, hamstrings, and the lower back.

Sets: 3 or 4

Reps: 10 to 12

Load: To be determined

Tempo: 3-0-1-0

Rest interval: Up to 15 seconds

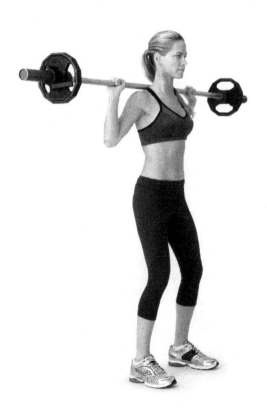
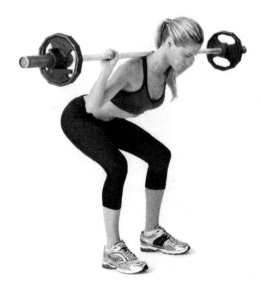

START POSITION

STAND straight with a bar resting across your upper back and your feet spaced hip-width apart.

THE MOVEMENT

BEND your knees slightly and pivot your torso forward from the hips until your upper body is almost parallel to the floor.

RETURN to the start position. Repeat to complete the set.

TIPS

THE range of motion in this exercise depends on the flexibility of your hamstrings. Lower the bar to your comfort level.

MAKE sure to maintain the arch in your lower back to avoid injuring it.

A4: Standing Split-Stance High-Pulley Face Pull

LOCATION: GYM

This exercise targets the muscles of your posterior shoulders and mid back (rhomboids and lower back).

Sets: 3 or 4

Reps: 10 to 12

Load: To be determined

Tempo: 3-0-1-0

Rest interval: Up to 15 seconds

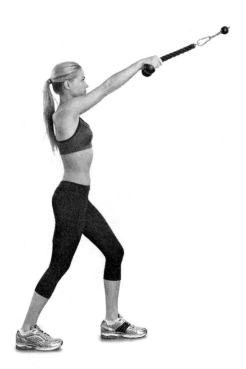
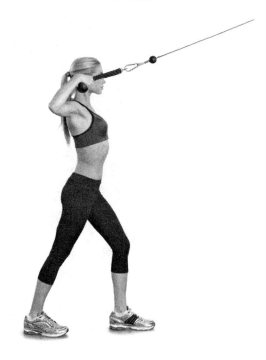

START POSITION

ATTACH a rope handle to a high-cable pulley.

GRIP the handle with your palms facing the floor. Take a few steps back and assume a split stance.

THE MOVEMENT

WITH your elbows held high, slowly pull the handle toward the lower part of your face (about eye level).

RETURN to the start position. Repeat to complete the set.

TIP

FOCUS on bringing your shoulder blades back and down, and keeping elbows at shoulder level.

A5: Dip

LOCATION: GYM

This exercise targets the triceps.

Sets: 3 or 4

Reps: 10 to 12

Load: Body weight

Tempo: 3-0-1-0

Rest interval: Up to 15 seconds

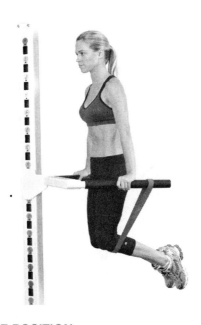
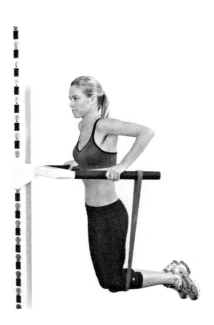

START POSITION

GRASP the handles of the dip station or dip assist machine and raise your body up, until your arms are completely straight. Use a grip slightly wider than the width of your body.

THE MOVEMENT

SLOWLY lower your body, keeping your elbows in at your sides, until your upper arms are parallel to the floor.

PUSH up to return to the start position. Repeat to complete the set.

TIPS

KEEP your torso as upright as possible; don't lean forward.

KEEP your elbows close to your body throughout the movement.

KEEP your core engaged throughout the movement.

IF this exercise is too challenging, use a band (as pictured) to help you.

A6: Hanging Knee Raise

LOCATION: GYM

This exercise targets the hip flexors and rectus abdominis.

Sets: 3 or 4

Reps: 10 to 12

Load: Body weight

Tempo: 2-0-2-0

Rest interval: Up to 120 seconds

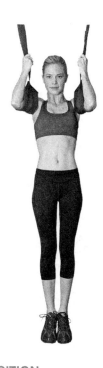
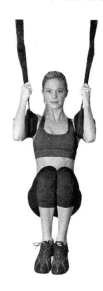

START POSITION

HANG from a pullup bar, hands shoulder-width apart, with your legs and feet together and your knees slightly bent. You may also use slinglike devices that attach to a bar, which allows you to place your upper arms inside them.

THE MOVEMENT

SLOWLY pull your knees up toward your chest while keeping your legs together. Think of curling your pelvis toward your chest as opposed to simply raising your legs.

RETURN to the start position. Repeat to complete the set.

TIP

TRY not to swing your body forward or backward, keeping your core tight as you raise and lower your body.

Energy System Training: Stationary Bike Plus Rowing Machine and/or VersaClimber

WEEK 1 (9 TO 15 MINUTES TOTAL), EST-13

WARMUP (stationary bike): 3 to 5 minutes, TBD, very low intensity

WORKOUT:

A: Stationary bike, 30 seconds of work (zones 4 to 5, RPE 7 to 10), followed by 60 seconds of recovery (zones 1 to 2, RPE 2 to 3); repeat 3 to 5 times

B: Rower or VersaClimber, 30 seconds of work (zones 4 to 5, RPE 7 to 10), followed by 60 seconds of recovery (zone 0, RPE 0); repeat 3 to 5 times

COOLDOWN (stationary bike): 3 to 5 minutes, TBD, very low intensity

WEEK 2 (10.5 TO 17.5 MINUTES TOTAL), EST-14

WARMUP (stationary bike): 3 to 5 minutes, TBD, very low intensity

WORKOUT:

A: Stationary bike, 45 seconds of work (zones 4 to 5, RPE 7 to 10), followed by 60 seconds of recovery (zones 1 to 2, RPE 2 to 3); repeat 3 to 5 times

B: Rower or VersaClimber, 45 seconds of work (zones 4 to 5, RPE 7 to 10), followed by 60 seconds of recovery (zone 0, RPE 0); repeat 3 to 5 times

COOLDOWN (stationary bike): 3 to 5 minutes, TBD, very low intensity

WEEK 3 (13.5 TO 18 MINUTES TOTAL), EST-15

WARMUP (stationary bike): 3 to 5 minutes, TBD, very low intensity

WORKOUT:

A: Stationary bike, 30 seconds of work (zones 4 to 5, RPE 7 to 10), followed by 60 seconds of recovery (zones 1 to 2, RPE 2 to 3); repeat 3 or 4 times

B: Rower or VersaClimber, 30 seconds of work (zones 4 to 5, RPE 7 to 10), followed by 60 seconds of recovery (zone 0, RPE 0); repeat 3 or 4 times

C: Stationary bike, 30 seconds of work (zones 4 to 5, RPE 7 to 10), followed by 60 seconds of recovery (zones 1 to 2, RPE 2 to 3); repeat 3 or 4 times

WEEK 4 (16 TO 21 MINUTES TOTAL), EST-16

WARMUP (stationary bike): 3 to 5 minutes, TBD, very low intensity

WORKOUT:

A: Stationary bike, 45 seconds of work (zones 4 to 5, RPE 7 to 10), followed by 60 seconds of recovery (stationary bike: zones 1 to 2, RPE 2 to 3); repeat 3 or 4 times

B: Rower or VersaClimber, 45 seconds of work (zones 4 to 5, RPE 7 to 10), followed by 60 seconds of recovery (zone 0, RPE 0); repeat 3 or 4 times

C: Stationary bike, 45 seconds of work (zones 4 to 5, RPE 7 to 10), followed by 60 seconds of recovery (zones 1 to 2, RPE 2 to 3); repeat 3 or 4 times

COOLDOWN (stationary bike): 3 to 5 minutes, TBD, very low intensity

EST RECOVERY SESSION (30 TO 45 MINUTES TOTAL), EST-R

WARMUP (stationary bike): 3 to 5 minutes, TBD, very low intensity

WORKOUT: Choose either treadmill, stationary bike, or elliptical (zone 2, RPE 3 to 4)

COOLDOWN (stationary bike): 3 to 5 minutes, TBD, very low intensity

ENERGY SYSTEM TRAINING POST-WORKOUT

FOAM rolling sequence (pages 42 to 45)

STATIC stretching (pages 45 to 47)

PHASE 4 NUTRITION
Phase 4 at a Glance

> **WEEKS 1 THROUGH 4**
>
> - Turn up your metabolic furnace.
> - Know your neurotransmitters.
> - Try carb cycling.
> - Support your thyroid with supplements.

You're 90 days into a healthier lifestyle. If you've followed the plan, you've seen a significant change in your physique by now—along with glowing skin, PMS-free periods, a higher libido, better energy levels, and increased self-esteem.

Some women, however, might follow this program to the letter but still struggle to shed body fat. Others may have lost a significant amount of body fat, only to now hit a plateau.

If this sounds like you—and you know you haven't slacked off on your program—your thyroid or brain chemistry could be the issue. The thyroid is your metabolic furnace, and your brain chemicals play an important part in weight loss, so you should consider them if your results are discouraging or your cravings have ramped up.

If your progress has been slow or you've hit a wall, Phase 4 can help push you through the plateau. (If you have slacked with the diet and exercise at all, tighten the reins—that's the quickest, easiest way to see better results.)

TURN UP YOUR METABOLIC FURNACE

If you are on thyroid medication, do not change your dose without supervision from your doctor—or find a new practitioner that can help you. That said, there are several things you can do to support your thyroid.

- **Give it a cold blast.** Finish your hot shower with a stimulating blast of cold water to the thyroid gland (the thyroid sits at the base of the neck, just above the collarbone).

- **Stoke the coals with coconut oil.** The medium-chain triglycerides in coconut oil make for extremely clean-burning fuel. Start with 1 to 2 tablespoons per day to help a sluggish metabolism. Cook with it (such as in sautés), or mix it into whey protein shakes or your high-fiber carb (tastes great with oat bran and mashed sweet potato). You'll find coconut oil at most health-food stores. (Also, www.tropicaltraditions.com is an excellent resource for coconut oil and coconut oil products, info, and recipes.)

- **Gulp some green tea.** Found in both caffeinated and decaffeinated green tea, the antioxidant EGCG (epigallocatechin gallate) stimulates the burning of fat. Don't care for tea? Try a high-quality EGCG supplement, such as Ultimate ECGC (Hardware).

- **Increase dietary iodine.** Sea veggies (such as seaweed and kelp), fish and shellfish, cow's-milk yogurt, low-fat mozzarella cheese, and strawberries are all good dietary sources of iodine. To keep iodine from being displaced in your body, thereby lowering thyroid function, do the following: Buy a water filter (see www.hightechhealth.com or www.doultonusa.com) that will remove the chlorine and fluoride from your tap water, and skip toothpastes with added fluoride. Use caution with "thyroid supportive" supplements, and only take iodine in supplement form with supervision.

- **Steer clear of heavy metals.** Heavy metals, particularly mercury (found in some dental fillings, fish, and vaccines), should be avoided as much as possible.

- **Reduce radiation.** Electromagnetic fields are everywhere in our modern world, from alarm clocks and cordless phones to microwaves and computers. The thyroid and its hormones are significantly impacted by EMF radiation.

- **Opt for organics.** Polychlorinated biphenyls and organochlorides in pesticides alter thyroid function and accumulate in body-fat tissue—both make it harder to lose fat.

- **Say no to soy.** Soy is the most problematic of the "goitrogens," a group of foods that also contains the Brassica family of vegetables (broccoli, cauliflower, cabbage, etc.). Minimize these vegetables if you have a thyroid condition, and avoid soy all together.

- **Skip wheat and dairy.** People with thyroid problems—particularly those with autoimmune thyroid issues—tend to be sensitive to dairy, wheat-based foods (breads, pasta, pastries, baked goods, beer, etc.), and other foods that contain the wheat protein gluten (such as oats, rye, couscous, Kamut, spelt, and teff).

KNOW YOUR NEUROTRANSMITTERS

These metabolic messengers in your brain and nervous system are important to cognitive processes such as concentration and to maintenance processes such as digestion and heart rate—and they can determine your cravings, too. In this phase, you'll support these pathways with diet, nutrition, and the timing of nutrients. Your reward: a brighter mood, more energy, and fewer cravings.

There are four main neurotransmitters to discuss: dopamine, acetylcholine, serotonin, and GABA (gamma-aminobutyric acid). For simplicity, let's categorize them as "uppers" and "downers" and focus on symptoms associated with low levels as they pertain to your cravings and mood.

YOUR UPPERS: BRAIN-ENERGIZING NEUROTRANSMITTERS

Dopamine

- **Responsible for:** Motivation and movement, excitement and energy, and pleasure

- **Deficiency can look like:** Fatigue, obesity, ADD, inability to concentrate, low libido, or depression (common in low-protein diets, particularly low animal-protein intake)

- **Low levels lead to:** Cravings for stimulants such as sugar, chocolate, caffeine, or alcohol

- **Boost levels with:** Foods that contain tyrosine, such as green leafy veggies, dairy, almonds, avocado, lima beans, pumpkin, and sesame seeds

Acetylcholine

- **Responsible for:** Processing speed, intellectual creativity, memory, and recollection of events, numbers, and names

- **Deficiency can look like:** Forgetfulness (forgetting phone numbers, where you put your keys or parked your car, etc.), burnout, paranoia, loss of creativity, or wanting to isolate (deficiencies common in low-fat diets)

- **Low levels lead to:** Cravings for fatty food, such as fried foods, pizza, cheese, ice cream, and cheesecake

- **Boost levels with:** Healthy fats, such as avocado and nuts, and choline-containing foods like whole eggs

YOUR DOWNERS: BRAIN-CALMING NEUROTRANSMITTERS

Serotonin

- **Responsible for:** Healthy digestion, joy, social engagement, and higher self-esteem

- **Deficiency can look like:** Insomnia, waking early or frequently during the night, IBS, PMS, aches and pains, sadness, depression, or anxiety

- **Low levels lead to:** Cravings for carbs, sugar, and salt; increased appetite in the later evening, particularly for carbs

- **Boost levels with:** Foods that contain tryptophan, such as turkey, sweet potato, cashews (most nuts and seeds), mango, and papaya

GABA

- **Responsible for:** Healthy digestion, sleep, relaxation, and tolerance of stress and pain

- **Deficiency looks like:** Anxiety, insomnia, increased sensitivity to pain, heartburn, headaches, irritable bowel syndrome, or emotional eating

- **Low levels lead to:** Emotional eating; overeating

- **Boost levels with:** Foods that contain glutamic acid, such as almonds, walnuts, halibut, whole oats, lentils, broccoli, spinach, and oranges

---

"carb pattern" to balance brain chemicals

To boost dopamine by day and increase serotonin in the evening, try carbohydrate patterning. This technique keeps these brain chemicals at the right levels at the right times of day and also keeps insulin low throughout the day.

Want to try it? Here's what to do.

- **For breakfast, lunch, and daytime snacks:** Avoid all carbs, with the exception of the fruit in your Recovery Shake. This keeps dopamine high when you want quick thinking and high energy.

- **For dinner and evening snacks:** Include a serving of high-fiber carbs to help raise serotonin levels. This will calm you and prep you for restful sleep. This also raises insulin, which lowers cortisol, and works well for those with insomnia.

TRY CARB CYCLING

Need to break through a plateau or budge some stubborn fat? A technique known as *carbohydrate cycling*—popular among bodybuilders—helps regulate leptin, the hormone that keeps hunger and cravings in check, and can give a boost to the thyroid.

There are various ways to cycle carbs to lose fat. This protocol depletes stored sugar in the liver and the muscles, which will really dip into fat stores. Here's what to do. Follow these instructions for 4-day intervals. After Day 4, repeat until desired results are achieved.

- **Days 1 and 2:** No carbs. This means no starches—whether Optimal, Allowable, or neither—and no fruit or honey in your Recovery Shake. Stick with lean protein and leafy green veggies. After your workout, mix up this no-carb Recovery Shake: 30 grams whey, 20 grams glycine, 20 grams glutamine, and 10 grams leucine (powdered amino acids will work best, but capsules are another option). Include a healthy-fat serving of ¼ cup of nuts, half an avocado, etc., with each meal.

- **Day 3:** No carbs; but boost amounts of healthy fats. For example, add ⅓ cup of nuts or avocado to each meal. Stick with above Recovery Shake recipe.

If you find 3 days of no carbs too daunting, substitute a low-carb day for Day 3, and spread 50 grams of carbs throughout your Recovery Shake, lunch, afternoon snack, and dinner. (Continue to skip carbs at breakfast.) Simply have 1 serving (4 bites) of fruit, sweet potato, whole oats, oat bran, or another Allowable carb for each of these meals and snacks.

- **Day 4:** High-carb day. You'll consume closer to 200 to 250 grams of carbs. On this day, you'll have a serving of Allowable carbs at every meal and snack, thus 5 times per day. For this day, bring fat intake back to normal (servings: 1 tablespoon of olive oil, half an avocado, ¼ cup or a small handful of nuts, etc.), and bring carb servings up to at least 6 bites or ½ cup. Consume at least 4 to 6 ounces of lean protein and liberal green veggies at each meal.

A FEW OTHER CONSIDERATIONS

- Add some recovery amino acids to your regimen to bolster your stamina—at least 300 milligrams of leucine, isoleucine, and valine (the branch-chain amino acids).

Consider 4 capsules of Ultimate Recovery Aminos (Hardware) twice daily between meals; take 1 dose post-workout.

- An alternative to carb cycling: Have 3 very low-carb days instead of no-carb days. In this version, have the Recovery Shake (without honey) with ½ cup of berries and a ½-cup serving of carbs at dinner, but avoid them the rest of the day.

- If your exercise performance suffers with a very low-carb intake, carb cycling may not be for you. Continue to follow the program, and accept that it will take you a bit longer to lose fat and that you may need to address adrenal or thyroid issues with a qualified practitioner.

SUPPORT YOUR THYROID WITH SUPPLEMENTS

- Selenium: 50 micrograms daily (consider a complete mineral blend, such as Complete Mineral Complex by Designs for Health), 1 capsule 3 times daily

- Zinc: Start with 30 milligrams daily, then dose according to the results of a zinc challenge test (for more information, visit www.bodybyhardware.com).

- Vitamin A: Ensure you do not exceed the RDA upper limit of 3,000 micrograms (10,000 IU) without supervision of a health-care provider, but know that deficiency is common.

- Omega-3 fatty acids: 2 to 6 grams per day

- *Coleus forskohlii*: 250 milligrams twice daily

- Holy basil: 400 milligrams daily

CHAPTER 12

What Now?

So here you are, at the end of the program. Presumably, you've lost fat, you look and feel fabulous, and you have improved your overall health. Your skin glows; your energy is through the roof; your mood is brighter; PMS or perimenopausal symptoms are greatly reduced or gone. If so, we're thrilled for you.

As we said from the beginning, on this program, there is no "end." The end of Phase 4 marks the beginning of the rest of your life, and you might as well live it as your Ultimate You.

> On this program, there is no "end."

Flip back to Chapter 1 and review your description of your Ultimate You. Have you made your vision a reality? Are you close? Do you have a ways to go? Regardless of your answer, give yourself some credit. You've accomplished a great deal.

You've learned to manipulate your hormones to lose fat, get fit, and improve your health.

You learned that the *quality* of the calories you take in is more important than the quantity and eat accordingly.

You've cleansed your environment of excess estrogens to get and stay lean—not to mention that you've decreased your risk of many health conditions.

Maybe you've reached goals that aren't related to fat loss—graduating from a half-pushup to a full pushup or feeling comfortable in a gym. (Don't knock them—these are significant accomplishments.)

Your next steps depend on whether you've reached your goals and are face to face with your Ultimate You or whether you still have a ways to go.

In a way, this chapter lays out "Phase 5," giving you nutritional strategies and training tips that will help you maintain your gains going forward—or help you close in on your Ultimate You.

Choose Track 1 if you've reached your goal. You'll learn how to extend and build on the successes of the past 4 months, so you can be fit and healthy for the rest of your life.

Choose Track 2 if you still have more fat to lose. You'll review core nutritional principles and learn a new workout scientifically proven to boost your metabolism into high gear.

Whichever track you choose, take a 1-week vacation from your workouts. A little loafing is good for the soul, and besides, your body needs the rest.

TRACK 1
If You've Reached Goal

Congratulations! Your hard work shows, in the mirror and on the scale. To document your new, fitter body, book a professional photo shoot, or simply snap some pictures at home. Either way, photos ensure that you'll never lose sight of your Ultimate You.

If fat loss is no longer your goal, what is? Do you want to take up a new sport? Enter a figure competition? Train for a half-marathon or even a triathlon?

NUTRITION PLAN

Since we're all unique, maintenance is different for everyone. We all have different amounts of carbs and calories that optimize weight loss and maintenance. But here are some general guidelines to keep you on the right path for life.

> Since we're all unique, maintenance is different for everyone.

- While you were on the program, you ate on plan 90 percent of the time. To maintain your new, fitter physique, loosen your reins slightly to 80 percent. At 80 percent, you might add 1 dairy or wheat serving per day (provided you are not allergic or sensitive to either food type); have a food you desperately missed, such as pasta, once a week; or occasionally have full-fat rather than low-fat cheese.

- If you are insulin resistant, stick to low-insulin breakfasts and smaller servings of carbs (i.e., 4 bites or ⅓ cup). If you're not, stick with your usual carb servings—⅓ to ½ cup, or 4 to 6 bites.

- If you feel deprived, add more carbs to your diet. Start by adding just 1 larger (½ cup) serving per day, watching for weight regain.

- If you've been eating very few carbs, add them back into your evening meal first.

- When in doubt, add back in fats before carbs. Translation: Be less concerned about the fat content of proteins, worry less about low-fat cheese or whether you eat a whole avocado versus a half, and continue to keep carbs in check.

- Set a "red alert" number over which your weight should not rise—5 to 7 pounds over your Ultimate You weight. Then weigh yourself once a week. If you hit that number, return to eating 90 percent on plan.

- Once a month, take your measurements and measure your percentage of body fat. Record them in a notepad you keep just for this purpose.

- Return to the Phase 1 supplement regimen of multivitamins, fish-oil capsules, and greens. After 3 months, switch it up.

  - Change your multivitamin for 1 month—for example, switch from Ultimate Metabolic Multi (Hardware) to Uber Nutrients from Poliquin Performance.

  - Change from high-dose omega-3 supplements to an omega blend (consider Omega Synergy from Designs for Health) for 1 month. Then return to 2 to 4 grams of omega-3 supplements daily for maintenance.

  - Take a break from greens for 1 month, so you won't develop sensitivities to their components.

  - Rotate your antioxidants. For example, if you are taking grapeseed extract, switch to resveratrol for 1 month.

  - Continue to rotate your supplement regimen every 3 months.

> Set a "red alert" number over which your weight should not rise—5 to 7 pounds over your Ultimate You weight. Then weigh yourself once a week. If you hit that number, return to eating 90 percent on plan.

---

reached your ultimate you?

We'd love to hear about it! Contact us via our Web site (www.bodybyhardware.com) with your success story. Include the "turning point" that led you to begin the program (a recent photo, a hurtful remark, a doctor-issued health warning, catching sight of your reflection in a mirror), your vision of your Ultimate You from Chapter 1, and your triumphs and struggles throughout each phase. Include your weight, body-fat percentage, and measurements before you started Phase 1 and after completing Phase 4, too. Your success will inspire others to take action, so pay it forward!

- Continue to manage or treat any particular hormonal issues you may have (for example, estrogen dominance or insulin resistance).
- Continue to enjoy your weekly splurge meal.

WORKOUT PLAN

1. STRENGTH TRAINING: Perform 2 circuits of the following: Select a) any 3 dynamic warmups, b) any 2 activation drills, and c) 5 or 6 exercises from Phase 2, 3, or 4. Perform them in a circuit 3 or 4 times, resting 30 to 60 seconds between each set and 2 minutes between each circuit. *Note:* Make sure you alternate between lower- and upper-body movements in your self-designed program. Also, always finish with foam rolling and static stretching.

2. EST: Perform EST 3 times a week, cycling between high-intensity, medium-intensity, and low-intensity sessions. Start all sessions with a 3- to 5-minute warmup and cooldown.

- **High-intensity session (bike or outdoor running):** 20 to 30 seconds of work (zone 5, RPE 9 to 10), followed by 60 to 90 seconds of recovery (zone 2, RPE 3 to 4). Repeat 6 to 8 times. *Note:* If you choose the 20-second work interval, use the 60-second recovery interval. If you opt for the 30-second work interval, take 90 seconds of rest.
- **Medium-intensity session (treadmill, bike, or outdoor running):** 120 to 180 seconds of work (zone 4, RPE 7 to 8), followed by 60 to 90 seconds

of recovery (zone 2, RPE 3 to 4); repeat 4 to 5 times. *Note:* If you choose the 180-second work interval, use the 90-second recovery interval. If you opt for the 120-second work interval, take 60 seconds of rest.

- **Low-intensity session:** Jog, cycle, swim, or perform another cardiovascular workout for 30 to 45 minutes in zones 2 to 3.

choosing a personal trainer

Want to push your training to the next level? Need extra motivation to reach goal? Either way, a personal trainer can help. But to find a good one, you need to know what to look for. Before you hire one, ask him or her the following questions.

■ **Are you certified or accredited?** A personal trainer should be certified through a reputable personal-training organization. Higher-level certifications include:

NSCA-CPT and CSCS (National Strength and Conditioning Association Certified Personal Trainer and Certified Strength and Conditioning Specialist)

ACSM CPT (American College of Sports Medicine)

NASM CPT (National Academy of Sports Medicine)

Continuing education certifications should come in addition to (not in place of) the above.

■ **How long have you been a personal trainer?** Ask how many years of experience a personal trainer has working with clients—he or she should have done so at least 1 year, as well as have worked with a broad range of clients—most importantly, clients similar to you, with your needs or limitations.

■ **What's your educational background?** While certification is the must-have credential, a college degree in exercise physiology or biomechanics is a plus. If the trainer doesn't have one, ask if he or she has taken basic courses in exercise physiology, biomechanics, kinesiology, and anatomy.

■ **Can you work with me on my nutrition program?** The trainer should have a BS or MS in nutrition, in addition to a personal training certificate, if he or she will be advising you on nutrition.

Ask the trainer if you can talk with a few former clients. Ask them if they were satisfied with their training and results; whether the trainer was professional, on time, and prepared; and whether their needs were addressed. If you hear good things, "audition" the trainer for a week or two to make sure that your personalities and goals mesh.

TRACK 2

If You're Not Quite There

First off, don't sweat it. Either your goal wasn't achievable (you can't lose 100 pounds in 4 months no matter what!) or your metabolism was damaged by years of misguided diets and needs more time to heal. The Chinese philosopher Confucius said, "When it is obvious that the goals cannot be reached, don't adjust the goals, adjust the action steps." That's what Track 2 is all about: tweaking your program.

> When it is obvious that the goals cannot be reached, don't adjust the goals, adjust the action steps.

We're confident that the nutritional and training strategies below will increase your body's ability to burn fat. To shake things up even more, hire a personal trainer (see page 253 for guidelines) or contact us through our Web site to get a custom plan.

NUTRITION PLAN

1. **Get back to basics.**

   - Continue to stay on plan 90 percent of the time, choosing most of your foods from the Optimal list.

   - Drink an adequate amount of water.

   - Manage your carbs; stick with the smaller portions (⅓ cup/4 bites).

   - Eat at least 4 ounces of protein per meal.

   - Eat hormone-free protein as much as possible. If you eat more than three meals per week away from home, eating more "clean" protein can help.

   - Continue to enjoy your splurge meal. If you've been skipping it in hopes of losing weight faster, reinstate it. Make sure the meal includes some starchy carbs to reset leptin and thyroid hormones.

   - If you drink alcohol more than once a week, cutting back can help you lose weight. At the very least, switch to clear, nonsugary mixed drinks and wine.

   - Return to the Phase 1 supplement regimen of multivitamins, fish-oil capsules, and greens.

- Continue to manage or treat any particular hormonal issues you may have (for example, estrogen dominance).

2. Step it up a notch.

- If you didn't try the modifications in the program, such as the low-insulin breakfasts and carb cycling, give them a go now.

- Keep a diet diary. It will keep you honest (yes, "tastes" and "bites" count) and help you identify and correct situations that derail your progress—doughnuts at the office, bingeing under stress, nibbling out of boredom, and so forth.

- Keep your diet clean, and tighten it where you can. You should already be eating mostly from the Optimal list, but also watch for dairy or a less-than-optimal protein choice, such as non-grass-fed steak, sneaking into your diet.

- Consider being evaluated by a nutritional medicine practitioner, so he or she can better target and treat any hormonal imbalances.

WORKOUT PLAN

1. STRENGTH TRAINING

- Repeat Phase 3, but add a fourth set. Keep rest periods as short as possible, and reduce rest between each circuit by 30 seconds.

2. EST

- Twice a week, perform 1 set of the Tabata Protocol (page 256).

- Optional: Follow the Tabata Protocol with 20 to 30 minutes of steady-state cardio.

- If you don't already, walk 60 minutes 5 or 6 times per week, preferably fasting, first thing in the morning.

---

switch it up!

Whether you're at goal or closing in on it, change your workout every 4 weeks. Keeping up that metabolic disturbance has several benefits: You'll be continually challenged, avoid muscular imbalances and injuries, and keep your body from adapting to a routine too easily, which is the primary cause of plateaus.

THE TABATA PROTOCOL

Track 2 takes the cardio up a notch. This high-intensity interval training (HIIT) routine burns *mucho* fat—and takes less than 15 minutes a *week*.

Named after Izumi Tabata, Ph.D., a former researcher at Japan's National Institute of Fitness and Sports in Kanoya, this protocol has you alternate between 20 seconds of intense exercise and 10 seconds of rest. Studies show that the protocol burns just as much fat as moderate aerobic workouts done for 45 minutes and keeps your metabolism revving for hours after you're finished.

If possible, perform Tabata on a Spin bike or rowing machine, or running on grass or on a Woodway Force treadmill—better yet, alternate among these.

One round of Tabata takes 12 to 14 minutes, including the warmup and cooldown. (Don't be discouraged if you have a difficult time doing this workout, as it taxes even professional athletes.)

- WARM UP FOR 3 TO 5 MINUTES. Start at a low intensity, and gradually increase it over the course of the warmup. Then continue to the intervals.

- WORK FOR 3 TO 5 MINUTES. For 20 seconds, go full speed as fast as you can. For the next 10 seconds, go slow. Continue this back-and-forth sequence for 4 minutes (8 intervals).

- RECOVER FOR 3 TO 5 MINUTES. After 8 intervals, depending on your method of choice, pedal, walk, or row slowly for 3 to 5 minutes.

Appendix

Training Log

Phase: _____ Date: _____ Name: _____

Target Date: _____ Mantra: _____

SEQ	WK	EXERCISE	SETS	REPS	TEMPO	REST	SET 1	SET 2	SET 3	SET 4
							load/reps lb/kg	load/reps lb/kg	load/reps lb/kg	load/reps lb/kg

Diet Diary

Ultimate You Diet Diary   Date: _____   Name: _____

Goal: Target Date: _____   Mantra: _____

TIME	FOOD AND DRINK INTAKE	P	F	RANK	WHY I CHOSE THIS	BOWEL & URINE	HOW I FELT (BOTH PHYSICALLY AND EMOTIONALLY)
6 a.m.							
7 a.m.							
8 a.m.							
9 a.m.							
10 a.m.							
11 a.m.							
12 a.m.							
1 p.m.							
2 p.m.							
3 p.m.							
4 p.m.							
5 p.m.							
6 p.m.							
7 p.m.							
8 p.m.							
9 p.m.							
Other				Day Rank			

Training Log and Diet Diary are available for download at www.bodybyhardware.com.

HOW TO USE THE DIET DIARY

- Simply write down what you eat and drink at the time you consume it. (This will help you fine-tune meal-timing intervals.)

- For the columns labeled "P" and "F," check the P column if you included a lean, high-quality protein and the F column if you included a fibrous veggie.

- Rank your adherence to the plan on a scale of 1 to 10, keeping track of every time you eat an item that's off plan (e.g., a packet of regular sugar in your coffee, a sugary condiment like ketchup or other sauce, a piece of bread). Each of those count as 1; for example, a lunch with an open-faced turkey sandwich on a baguette (unallowed carb) or an omelet with broccoli and Cheddar cheese (unallowed fat). For a perfectly on-plan meal, assign a zero.

- The end of the "Rank" column is the "Day Rank." To get this number, add up your numbers in the Rank column and subtract from 10. This is your "X /10" for the day. If you are frequently below 8/10 (i.e., more than twice per week), tighten up the diet to keep losing. Remember, for fat loss, you are aiming for 90 percent adherence, and for maintenance, you are aiming for 80 percent adherence to the plan.

- Your splurge meal does not count in this numbering system—that is a freebie!

- To troubleshoot challenges that can derail your ability to stay on plan, answer the following questions each time you choose an off-plan food.

Did you eat it to indulge a craving?

Did you eat it because you were hungry? Ravenous?

Did you eat it because you were low in energy?

If you answered yes to any of the above, check your food diary and examine your previous meal.

Did it contain protein? Fibrous veggies? If not, add them into your next meal and ask the same questions. If yes, increase both at your next meal.

Did it include a high-fiber carb? If not and you answered yes to any of the questions above, add 4 to 6 bites of a high-fiber carb to your next meal and reassess. If you were very low in energy, be sure to eat every 3 hours to keep your blood sugar up.

Are you drinking enough water? Typically, 3 to 5 liters is enough for most women.

To know if a meal agreed with you, answer the questions below when you've finished eating.

How is your sense of well-being? Is it low or "off"?

Do you feel sleepy?

Do you have any digestive upset—bloating, excessive fullness, diarrhea?

If you answered yes to any of the above:

Eat more slowly, and consider a digestive enzyme formula such as Ultimate Digestizymes.

Ensure that your carbs were from the Optimal list for high-fiber starches.

Use your food journal to track which proteins best agree with you. You may find that you feel best on grass-fed beef rather than chicken or that you do well on fatty fish like salmon.

If you are feeling sleepy after a meal, be sure to utilize Phase 2 supplements, particularly the Ultimate Insulin Manager.

Are you drinking enough water? Typically, 3 to 5 liters is enough for most women.

To know if a meal agreed with you, answer the questions below when you've finished eating.

How is your sense of well-being? Is it low or "off"?

Do you feel sleepy?

Do you have any digestive upset—bloating, excessive fullness, diarrhea?

If you answered yes to any of the above:

Eat more slowly, and consider a digestive enzyme formula such as Ultimate Digestizymes.

Ensure that your carbs were from the Optimal list for high-fiber starches.

Use your food journal to track which proteins best agree with you. You may find that you feel best on grass-fed beef rather than chicken or that you do well on fatty fish like salmon.

If you are feeling sleepy after a meal, be sure to utilize Phase 2 supplements, particularly the Ultimate Insulin Manager.

The Ultimate You
Food-Label Decoder

THERE ARE VERY FEW BAGGED or boxed items on the Ultimate You plan. At some point, however, you'll have to decipher nutritional labels on packaged foods—and we do mean decipher, since the labels can be misleading. Here's what you need to know.

- Ingredients on labels are usually listed by weight, from the highest volume to lowest volume.

- Portion sizes are based on a standardized reference that is often less than what we normally choose here in our "supersized" world. What the label lists as the portion size may not equal your reality; be sure to read the fine print.

- Be on the lookout for the truly "bad fats": partially hydrogenated oils. Avoid these at all costs. Stick with extra-virgin olive oil, coconut oil, avocado, cold-water fish, and raw nuts and seeds as your principal sources of fat.

- Natural doesn't necessarily equal healthy. Many people walk into a health-food store assuming everything there is healthy. A cookie is still a cookie, even if it's vegan, gluten free, and sweetened with agave syrup. It's not that all healthy versions of desserts and other foods are outright terrible, but any processed food lacks fiber and thus is worse for fat loss. Further, any food sweetened with anything other than sugar alcohol or an artificial sweetener will raise insulin.

- Technically, a product needs to have 95 percent organic ingredients to put "organic" as part of the product name. For more details, see the USDA Web site: http://www.ams.usda.gov.

- Not all foods are required to include labeling information. The exceptions: fresh supermarket food such as raw fruits, vegetables, fish, meat and poultry products (unless they are processed), and restaurant foods—although some places, like New York City, are beginning to require restaurants to disclose pertinent nutritional information. Whatever the case, don't let ignorance be an excuse for unhealthy choices—read your labels and investigate.

SYNONYMS FOR SUGAR

Sugar has many "aliases." Some you know: brown sugar, confectioner's sugar, honey, molasses or blackstrap molasses, and maple syrup. Regardless of name, *all* sugar causes an insulin response. Here are more aliases, so you're not fooled by "natural" sugars or hidden sources.

- Agave
- Barley malt
- Brown rice syrup
- Cane sugar
- Corn sweetener
- Corn syrup
- Date sugar
- Dextrin
- Dextrose
- D-mannose
- Evaporated cane juice
- Fruit juice concentrate
- Glucose
- High-fructose corn syrup (HFCS)
- Invert sugar
- Lactose
- Maltodextrin
- Maltose
- Malt syrup
- Raw sugar
- Sucanat
- Sucrose
- Turbinado sugar

ALLOWABLE CLAIMS ON LABELS

You may see the claims below that are "guidelines" for making healthy choices.

1. ***Eating enough calcium may help prevent osteoporosis.***
   Green, leafy veggies are great sources of calcium.

2. ***Limiting the amount of sodium you eat may help prevent hypertension.***
   True, but it's important to note that not all hypertension is sodium related.

3. ***Limiting the amount of saturated fat and cholesterol you eat may help prevent heart disease.***
   Be mindful that saturated fat is just one factor in heart disease and that some saturated fats, like coconut oil, do not contribute to poor health.

4. *Eating fruits, vegetables, and grain products that contain dietary fiber may help prevent heart disease.*

   This is why oatmeal can claim it lowers cholesterol. However, it's best to get your fiber from vegetables and fruits, rather than high amounts of grains.

5. *Limiting the amount of total fat you eat may help reduce your risk of cancer.*

   All fats are not created equal; some types are healthier than others, and low-fat diets can be very unhealthy.

6. *Eating fiber-containing grain products, fruits, and vegetables may help prevent cancer.*

   The best starchy fiber sources are sweet potatoes, yams, pumpkin, winter squashes, and legumes, followed by sprouted-grain products and whole grains like oats, quinoa, and brown rice.

7. *Eating fruits and vegetables that are low in fat and good sources of dietary fiber, vitamin A, or vitamin C may help prevent cancer.*

   The fiber and array of phytonutrients and antioxidants in plant foods make them truly outstanding.

KNOW THE LINGO: WHAT THESE TERMS MEAN

Dietary Fiber

- *High-fiber:* 5 grams of fiber or more per serving
- *A good source of fiber:* 2.5 to 4.9 grams of fiber per serving

Fat

- *Fat-free:* Less than ½ gram of fat per serving
- *Low-fat:* 3 grams of fat or less per serving
- *Lean:* Less than 10 grams of fat, less than 4½ grams of saturated fat, and no more than 95 milligrams of cholesterol per serving
- *Extra-lean:* Less than 5 grams of fat, less than 2 grams of saturated fat, and no more than 95 milligrams of cholesterol per serving

- *Low in saturated fat:* 1 gram of saturated fat or less per serving and no more than 15 percent of calories from saturated fatty acids

- *Reduced* or *less fat:* At least 25 percent less fat per serving than the higher-fat version

Cholesterol

- *Low cholesterol:* 20 milligrams of cholesterol or less and 2 grams of saturated fat or less per serving

- *Reduced cholesterol:* At least 25 percent less cholesterol than the higher-cholesterol version and 2 grams or less of saturated fat per serving

- *Cholesterol-free:* Less than 2 milligrams of cholesterol or 2 grams or less of saturated fat per serving

Sugar

- *Sugar-free:* Less than ½ gram of sugar per serving

- *Low sugar:* May not be used as a claim

- *Reduced sugar:* At least 25 percent less sugar per serving, compared with a similar food

- *No added sugars, without added sugar,* or *no sugar added*: No amount of sugar or any other ingredient that contains sugars that functionally substitutes for added sugars is added during processing or packaging; the product contains no ingredients that contain added sugars, such as jam, jelly, or concentrated fruit juice

Calories

- *Calorie-free:* Fewer than 5 calories per serving

- *Low calorie:* 40 calories or less per serving

- *Light* or *"lite"*: Less calories or no more than half the fat of the higher-calorie, higher-fat version

- *Reduced calorie:* At least 25 percent fewer calories per serving, compared with a similar food

Sodium (goal: 2,400 mg or less per day)

- *Light in sodium:* No more than half the sodium of the higher-sodium version

- *Sodium-free:* Less than 5 milligrams of sodium per serving and no sodium chloride (NaCl) in ingredients

- *Very low sodium:* 35 milligrams of sodium or less per serving

- *Low sodium:* 140 milligrams of sodium or less per serving

- *Reduced* or *less sodium:* 25 percent less sodium per serving than the higher-sodium version

Descriptive Terms You Should Know

- *Free:* Contains the least amount of an ingredient; *very low* and *low* have slightly more

- *Reduced* or *less:* Contains 25 percent less of that nutrient than the reference version of that food

- *Good source of:* Contains 10 to 19 percent of the Daily Value (DV) per serving. *Note:* Daily Value is often much lower than what the Ultimate You plan recommends.

- *High, rich in,* or *excellent source of:* Contains 20 percent or more of the DV per serving (these are better choices than *good source of*)

- *More, fortified, enriched,* or *added:* Contains at least 10 percent more of the DV for protein, vitamins, minerals, or fiber per serving

- *Fresh:* Has not been frozen, heat-processed, or similarly processed

LABEL MATH

To assess a packaged food for balance in terms of proteins and carbs, subtract the grams of fiber from the total carbohydrate number. (Since fiber does not affect blood sugar levels, you don't count fiber grams as carbs.) This number should be in proportion to the protein number.

For example, the label on Kashi GoLean cereal says 1 serving contains 23 grams of total carbohydrate and 8 grams of fiber, making the total carb load on your blood sugar 15 grams. This is in proportion to 1 serving's 10 grams of protein, as the ratio is 3 to 2 of carbs to protein. Thus, this would be a good choice if you wanted to have packaged cereal.

By contrast, 1 serving of Grape-Nuts cereal contains 47 grams of total carbohydrate and 5 grams of fiber, leaving 42 grams of net carbs. Since 1 serving contains 6 grams of protein, its ratio of carbs to protein is 7 to 1, which is out of proportion.

Cereals in general are not a great choice, as they are highly processed and typically too high in carbs. High-protein cereals generally contain significant amounts of soy protein, which is not recommended for every woman and can cause substantial gas and bloating. Better choices for high-fiber starches are legumes, sprouted-grain breads, root vegetables, and squashes.

Recommended Supplements by Phase

All supplements are Hardware brand unless otherwise noted; all Designs for Health and Hardware products available at www.bodybyhardware.com.

PHASE 1

- Ultimate Metabolic Multi: 2 with meals, 3 times daily

- Ultimate Omega 3: 1 or 2 with meals, 3 times daily

- Ultimate Greens: 1 tablespoon twice daily in water

    OR

- Ultimate Antiox, Resveratrol Synergy (Designs for Health)/GrapeSeed Supreme (Designs for Health): 1 to 3 capsules per day or as directed on bottle

PHASE 2

- Ultimate CLA: 2 with meals, 3 times daily

- Ultimate Insulin Manager: 1 to 3 capsules with all meals and snacks (titrate up your dose by one cap each time)

- Ultimate Fiber: 1 tablespoon 1 to 5 times daily in water

- Ultimate Fat Burner: 2 or 3 with meals, 3 times daily

- Zinc Supreme (Designs for Health): 1 or more capsules daily (determine dose via zinc challenge)

- MagneDerm (Designs for Health) OR Topical Mag (Poliquin Performance): $\frac{1}{4}$ to $\frac{1}{2}$ teaspoon applied topically to arms or legs, 1 to 4 times daily

PHASE 3

- Grapeseed Supreme (Designs for Health) OR Resveratrol Synergy (Designs for Health): 1 with meals, 3 times daily

- Ultimate Liquid Carnitine: 1 or 2 teaspoons, 1 to 3 times daily

- Libido Stim F (Designs for Health): 1 or 2 with meals, 3 times daily

PHASE 4

- Complete Mineral Complex (Designs for Health): 1 capsule, 3 times daily with food

Ultimate You 1-Week Optimal Menu with Low-Insulin Breakfasts and 5 p.m. Workouts

- The menu on page 272 is assembled completely from choices on the Optimal list: 3 meals and 2 snacks spaced evenly at 3- to 4-hour intervals.

- Follow specifically, or use this menu as a template to plan your workouts and meals.

- Workouts can always be done morning, afternoon, or evening; count your Recovery Shake as 1 snack for the day.

- Four to 6 bites of Optimal high-fiber starch or 1 serving Optimal fruit choice is allowed at any meal, although breakfast options are specifically no carb (i.e., they are low-insulin breakfast options for those with insulin resistance; see Phase 2).

- Do not use a Recovery Shake after recovery sessions or on days off from exercise.

- If you are not following the low-insulin protocol, add high-fiber carbs to any meal (4 to 6 bites per serving).

- If you are following the low-insulin protocol, do not eat carbs at breakfast; however, be sure to include a serving of fat (e.g., ¼ cup nuts).

Ultimate You 1-Week Optimal Menu with
Low-Insulin Breakfasts and 5 p.m. Workouts

	MONDAY	TUESDAY	WEDNESDAY	THURSDAY	FRIDAY	SATURDAY	SUNDAY
Breakfast	Mushroom & Spinach Scramble (pg 275)	Bell Pepper Boats (pg 277)	Greek Eggs (pg 275)	Smoked Salmon sans Bagel (pg 276)	BT Eggs (pg 275)	3 Simple Poached Eggs (pg 276), 1 c blanched spinach	Veggie Frittata (pg 276)
Mid-morning Snack	½ c Guacamole (pg 288), sliced bell pepper wedges	Celery sticks, 2 tsp nut butter	½ bison burger, 1 small sliced tomato	2 Spinach Timbales (pg 287), ¼ c nuts	1–2 Grass-Fed Meat Muffins (pg 284), 1 c cucumber slices	1 can salmon or trout, 10 asparagus spears	4 Slentiva chews
Lunch	Greek Salad (pg 278) served w/grilled chicken	(leftover) Spicy Bison-n-Kale Chipotle Chili over spinach	Coconut Cinnamon Chicken (pg 283) over spinach or w/mixed green salad	(leftover) Fajita-Style Shrimp over spinach	Smoked Salmon & Avocado Wrap (pg 280)	Lemon Walnut Chicken Salad (pg 279)	Shrimp Marinara (pg 281) w/mixed green salad
Mid-afternoon Snack	None	Ultimate You Lean Bar	None	Apple, ¼ c nuts	None	1 slice Veggie Frittata (pg 276)	1 can sardines, ½ c raspberries
EXERCISE 5 p.m.	Strength training	EST	Strength training	EST	Strength training	Recovery session	Day off
Post-Workout (counts as 1 snack)	Recovery Shake (pg 37)	None	Recovery Shake (pg 37)	None	Recovery Shake (pg 37)	None	None
Dinner	Bison-n-Kale Chipotle Chili (pg 283) over spinach	Baked Salmon & Red Swiss Chard (pg 284)	Fajita-Style Shrimp (pg 282) over spinach	Grass-Fed Meat Loaf (pg 284) w/mixed green salad	Green Beans & Almond Chicken (pg 281)	Splurge meal!	Asian Chicken Stir-Fry (pg 281)

Ultimate You 1-Week Allowable Menu with Morning Workouts

- The menu on page 274 includes Optimal and Allowable choices; 3 meals and 2 snacks spaced evenly at 3- to 4-hour intervals.

- Follow specifically, or use this menu as a template to plan your workouts and meals.

- Workouts can always be done morning, afternoon, or evening; count Recovery Shake as one snack for the day.

- Four to 6 bites of an Optimal or Allowable high-fiber starch or 1 serving of an Optimal or Allowable fruit choice is allowed at any meal; suggestions are included, but substitute as you wish.

- Only use a Recovery Shake after strength-training sessions.

- If you are not following the low-insulin protocol, add high-fiber carbs to any meal (4 to 6 bites per serving).

- If you are following the low-insulin protocol, do not eat carbs at breakfast; however, be sure to include a serving of fat (e.g., ¼ cup nuts).

Ultimate You 1-Week Allowable Menu with Morning Workouts

	MONDAY	TUESDAY	WEDNESDAY	THURSDAY	FRIDAY	SATURDAY	SUNDAY
EXERCISE (first thing in morning)	Strength training	EST	Strength training	EST	Strength training	Recovery session or day off	Day off
Post-Workout (counts as 1 snack)	Recovery Shake w/1 scoop whey & ½ c berrie	None	Recovery Shake w/1 scoop whey & ½ c berries	None	Recovery Shake w/1 scoop whey & ½ c berries	None	None
Breakfast	Turkey BLT (pg 277), ½ c oat bran made with water (optional)	Mexi-Eggs (pg 276), ½ c black beans (optional)	Asparagus & Mushroom Scramble (pg 275) w/low-fat Swiss, 4–6 bites hemp bread toast (optional)	Pesto Toast & Eggs (pg 278)	1 c Greek yogurt w/Not-Granola (pg 287), ½ c blueberries	Healthy Eggs Benedict (pg 277)	Veggie Frittata (pg 276)
Mid-morning Snack	None	Celery sticks with 2 tsp nut butter	None	Hard-boiled egg and ½ c berries	None	Ultimate You Bar	Pear, ¼ c nuts
Lunch	Artichoke & Hearts of Palm Salad w/grass-fed bison burger, 2 high-fiber crackers (optional)	(leftover) Cashew Chicken Curry over Spinach	(leftover) Apricot Cod w/mixed green salad, 2 high-fiber crackers (optional)	Steak & Arugula Salad (pg 279) w/shaved Parmesan	(leftover) Coconut Green Curry Chicken Meat Loaf w/ Cucumber Pear Salad	Turkey burger w/mixed green salad, ½ c Lentil Salad (optional, pg 285)	(leftover) Laura's Hearty Tuscan Soup over spinach, 2 high-fiber crackers (optional)
Mid-afternoon Snack	Sliced bell pepper wedges w/2 oz goat cheese	1 hard-boiled egg, ¼ c Spicy Nut Mix (pg 288)	1 Cocoa Coconut PB Protein No-Bake Cookie (pg 287)	Apple w/2 tsp natural nut butter	2 oz dark chocolate	2 high-fiber crackers w/2 oz goat cheese	Warm Berry Compote (pg 288)
Dinner	Cashew Chicken Curry (pg 282) over spinach	Apricot Cod (pg 282) w/steamed asparagus or mixed green salad	Mango Chicken (pg 281) over spinach, ½ c Spicy Black beans (optional, pg 285)	Coconut Green Curry Chicken Meat Loaf (pg 284), Cucumber Pear Salad (pg 279)	Splurge meal!	Laura's Hearty Tuscan Soup (pg 282) over spinach, 4–6 bites sprouted-grain garlic toast (optional)	Sausage & Pepper Stir-Fry, ½ c Tapas-Style Chickpeas (optional, pg 285)

Ultimate You Meals

- All meal options are "Optimal" unless labeled as "Allowable."
- Unless otherwise noted, all recipes serve one.
- *Interchangeable*: Tired of eggs? Try something you normally think of as lunch fare for breakfast.

BREAKFAST
Quick Scrambles and More

Mushroom & Spinach

Sauté 1 cup mushrooms and 1 cup spinach in 1 tablespoon olive oil for 2 minutes. Add 3 eggs or 5 egg whites. Season with sea salt and pepper. (Allowable option: 1 tablespoon goat cheese.)

Greek Eggs

Sauté 1 small diced tomato and 1 cup spinach with 1 teaspoon chopped fresh garlic or ¼ teaspoon garlic powder and both sea salt and pepper to taste in 1 tablespoon olive oil for 2 minutes. Add 3 eggs or 5 egg whites. (Allowable option: 1 tablespoon feta cheese.)

BT (Broccoli & Turkey) Eggs

Sauté 1 cup chopped broccoli florets and 1 ounce sliced turkey in 1 tablespoon olive oil for 2 to 3 minutes. Add 3 eggs or 5 egg whites. (Allowable option: 1 tablespoon goat cheese or 1 ounce low-fat Swiss cheese.)

Asparagus & Mushroom

Sauté ½ cup sliced mushrooms and 1 cup chopped asparagus in 1 tablespoon olive oil for 2 to 3 minutes. Add 3 eggs or 5 egg whites. Season with sea salt and pepper. (Optional: Add 1 ounce low-fat Swiss cheese.)

Green Eggs

Sauté 1 cup spinach in 1 tablespoon olive oil. Add 3 eggs or 5 egg whites. When eggs are nearly cooked, add 1 tablespoon basil pesto (add pesto near end to avoid burning it).

Mexi-Eggs

Scramble 3 eggs or 5 egg whites with spinach. Top with ⅓ cup fresh salsa and ½ avocado. (For non-low-insulin plan, serve with ½ cup black beans.)

Simple Poached Eggs

Serve 3 poached eggs (season as desired) alongside spinach salad made with olive oil and balsamic vinegar. If desired, add ½ cup diced tomato and/or ½ cup sliced cucumbers, or serve with 1 to 2 cups steamed greens of your choice.

Smoked Salmon sans Bagel

Serve 4 ounces smoked salmon with 1 cup (or more) sliced cucumbers and ½ cup sliced strawberries.

Smoked Salmon & Avocado Wrap

Lay 4 ounces smoked salmon and ½ avocado in 3 washed romaine leaves. Sprinkle with black pepper, if desired, and top with another romaine leaf. Eat as a sandwich.

Veggie Frittata (makes 6 servings)

Mix 10 organic omega-3 eggs with 2 tablespoons milk or plain unsweetened almond milk. Place in fridge to cool while prepping other ingredients. Sauté 1 clove chopped garlic with 2 cubed portobello mushroom tops, ½ cup chopped scallions (include some green stems), and 1 bunch asparagus chopped in 1-inch pieces (use upper third of the stalks) in 3 tablespoons olive oil. Season with ¼ teaspoon sea salt, 1 teaspoon Italian seasoning blend, and pepper to taste. Cook for 5 minutes and reduce heat to low. (Allowable option: Add ½ cup feta cheese or grated low-fat Swiss cheese to egg mixture.) Add egg mixture; cover and cook for 10 minutes, or until eggs are set and no liquid remains.

VARIATIONS:
SUB VEGGIES WITH ANY OF THE FOLLOWING:

> 7-ounce can of diced green chilies (drained), 1 cup chopped bell pepper
>
> 1 cup broccoli florets, 1 chopped bell pepper, 3 slices crumbled turkey bacon
>
> 1 chopped bell pepper, 2 diced shallots, 2 tablespoons fresh chopped parsley

Bell Pepper Boats

Wash, halve, and clean out a bell pepper. Scramble 3 eggs or 5 egg whites; season as desired. Divide eggs in half; place half in each bell pepper half and eat like a sandwich. (Allowable option: Spread ½ tablespoon goat cheese or ½ tablespoon basil pesto on each bell pepper half before filling with eggs.)

Turkey BLT

Lay 4 slices turkey bacon and 1 small sliced Roma tomato in 3 or 4 washed romaine lettuce leaves. Top with 1 or more lettuce leaves and season with cracked black pepper to taste. (Allowable option: 1 tablespoon goat cheese.)

NOTES FOR QUICK SCRAMBLES AND MORE

- If you're following low-insulin protocol, add ¼ cup nuts or 2 teaspoons nut butter to the above meals (except those that include avocado); do not add cheese.

- If you are not following low-insulin protocol, it is okay to add 1 serving (⅓ to ½ cup or 4 to 6 bites) of an Allowable high-fiber starch or an Optimal fruit, if not otherwise listed.

- Green veggies should be eaten liberally. It's fine to go over the recommended amounts for any nonstarchy vegetable or to serve spinach or green salad aside any breakfast option.

Other Allowable Options

Healthy Eggs Benedict

Mix "sauce" together with a fork: 3 tablespoons low-fat ricotta cheese, ½ teaspoon fresh chopped rosemary, 1½ teaspoons avocado or olive oil, 1 tablespoon lemon juice, a dash of cayenne, and both sea salt and pepper to taste. Toast 1 slice hemp or sprouted-grain bread. Place 2 poached eggs atop toast and top with sauce. Note: For a veggie option, serve alongside a small green salad or scramble 2 eggs with spinach instead of poaching them.

Pesto Toast & Eggs

Spread 2 teaspoons basil pesto on 1 slice toasted hemp or sprouted-grain bread. Scramble 2 eggs with 1 cup spinach, onion, mushrooms, or other veggie and place on top of toast. Add slice of tomato if desired. Eat as open-faced sandwich.

Greek Yogurt with Not-Granola

Mix 1 cup low-fat Greek yogurt with ¼ cup Not-Granola mix (page 287) and ½ cup blueberries.

Quick Protein-n-Oatmeal Porridge

Stir ½ scoop whey protein powder into ½ cup cooked steel-cut oats or oat bran (made with water). Add any or all of the following as desired: ¼ cup berries, 2 tablespoons nuts, ½ teaspoon cinnamon, and xylitol, stevia, or erythritol to desired sweetness. Serve with 1 or 2 hard-boiled organic eggs.

Meal-Replacement Whey Protein Shake

Blend 1 scoop Ultimate Whey, ½ cup frozen berries, and 1 tablespoon nut butter or 1 tablespoon coconut oil with 2 tablespoons whole oats or 1 tablespoon Ultimate Fiber with ½ to 1 cup water or unsweetened almond milk.

LUNCH & DINNER

Salads

Greek Salad

Dress romaine lettuce or mixed greens with olive oil and balsamic vinegar. Add sliced tomato, diced purple onion if desired, and ¼ cup kalamata olives; season with Italian seasoning blend and add sea salt and pepper to taste. (Allowable option: Add 2 table-spoons feta cheese.) Add grilled chicken, grilled shrimp, or other lean protein.

Lemon Walnut Chicken Salad

Dress romaine lettuce with walnut oil and lemon juice and 1 small sliced tomato. Season with sea salt and cracked black pepper to taste. Top with ¼ cup whole walnuts and grilled chicken. (Allowable option: Add feta cheese.)

Romaine & Apple Salad

Dress romaine lettuce with olive oil and 1 teaspoon Dijon mustard. Season with sea salt, rosemary, and black pepper. Top with ½ cup diced green apple and 1 grilled chicken breast or baked fish fillet.

Artichoke & Hearts of Palm Salad

Dress mixed greens with olive oil and white balsamic vinegar. Add ¼ cup sliced artichoke hearts and ½ cup sliced hearts of palm. Top with 1 grilled skinless chicken breast or fish fillet.

Steak & Arugula Salad

Dress arugula with olive oil and lemon juice. Season with sea salt and pepper to taste. Top with 4 ounces thinly sliced grass-fed steak. (Allowable option: 2 ounces Parmesan shaved into wide strips.)

Cucumber Pear Salad

Toss 2 diced cucumbers and 2 pears cut into bite-size pieces with 1 tablespoon coconut oil and 2 tablespoons white wine vinegar. Add sea salt and black pepper to taste. (Note: Coconut oil will appear waxy once it returns to room temperature, but it adds a light coconut taste.) Serve with grilled chicken breast, steamed fish, or Coconut Green Curry Chicken Meat Loaf (page 284).

Tomato Basil Salad (2 servings)

Combine ½ cup chopped fresh basil with 1 to 2 diced heirloom or other variety tomatoes and 1 tablespoon olive oil. Season with sea salt and black pepper to taste. Serve with grass-fed beef burger, fish, or grilled chicken. (Note: This tastes even better after it sits for a while, so double or triple this recipe and serve with eggs the next morning, or have with a protein serving for lunch.)

Note: Any green or other veggie can become a salad by drizzling it with olive oil and balsamic vinegar, then seasoning with your favorite spices. Try using chopped bell peppers, sliced cucumbers, or steamed asparagus spears as "salad" ingredients to keep from getting bored with spinach and mixed greens. Aim for 2 cups of veggies at each meal.

Quick Options

Smoked Salmon & Avocado Wrap

Lay 4 ounces smoked salmon and ½ avocado in 3 washed romaine leaves. Sprinkle with black pepper if desired, and top with another romaine leaf. Eat as a sandwich.

Turkey BLT

Lay 4 slices turkey bacon and 1 small sliced Roma tomato in 3 or 4 washed romaine lettuce leaves. Top with 1 or more lettuce leaves and season with cracked black pepper to taste. (Allowable option: 1 tablespoon goat cheese.)

Bison or Grass-Fed Beef or Turkey Burger & Red Leaf Salad

Toss red leaf lettuce with olive oil and balsamic vinegar or lemon juice. Season with Italian seasoning, sea salt, and pepper to taste. Serve alongside grilled burger with a thick slice of beefsteak, heirloom, or Jersey tomato. (Optional: Top burger with 1 tablespoon goat cheese.) Perfect topping for burgers: Cut red onion into large rings. Sauté with 1 clove chopped garlic in 1 tablespoon olive oil; cook until onion softens.

Crab & Avocado Salad

Mix together 4 ounces cooked fresh crabmeat, ½ cup chopped celery, 1 teaspoon olive oil mayonnaise, 1 teaspoon cumin, ½ teaspoon turmeric, 1 tablespoon capers, juice of ½ lemon, and sea salt and pepper to taste. Serve over a bed of watercress and top with ½ sliced avocado.

Quick Pre-Prepped Protein & Veggies

Serve previously baked chicken breasts or grilled grass-fed beef, bison, or turkey burgers alongside previously steamed greens or asparagus spears.

Supereasy Stir-Fries, Sautés, and Simmers

All recipes are single servings unless otherwise indicated. They are easily doubled for cooking for more than one or for making leftovers for the next day.

Asian Chicken Stir-Fry

Sauté 1 clove chopped garlic and 1 cubed chicken breast in 1 tablespoon olive oil. When chicken is nearly done, add leaves of 1 to 2 cleaned baby bok choy, 1 cup shiitake mushrooms, ¼ cup fresh chopped cilantro, and a dash each of white pepper and sea salt to taste. Cook for 3 more minutes or until veggies start to change color.

Classic Chicken Stir-Fry

Sauté 1 clove chopped garlic and 1 cubed chicken breast in 1 tablespoon olive oil. When chicken is nearly done, add 1 cup broccoli florets, ½ cup diced celery, ½ cup sliced carrots, and ½ cup sliced mushrooms. Season with sea salt and pepper to taste. Cook for 3 more minutes, or until veggies start to change colors.

Green Beans & Almond Chicken

Sauté 1 clove chopped garlic and 1 diced chicken breast in 1 tablespoon olive oil. When chicken is nearly done, add 2 cups cleaned green beans (cut into 1- to 2-inch pieces) and ¼ cup almonds. Season with sea salt and pepper to taste. Cook for 3 more minutes, or until green beans start to change colors.

Mango Chicken (2 servings)

Sauté 2 cloves chopped garlic and 2 cubed chicken breasts in 2 tablespoons olive oil. When chicken is nearly done, add 1 cup chopped mushrooms, 1 thinly sliced mango, and 1 chopped onion. Add ½ teaspoon white pepper; season with sea salt to taste. Cook 3 more minutes, then add 1½ cups chunky fresh salsa (mango peach or pineapple mango varieties are often available; just watch for added sugar) and let simmer for 5 minutes. Serve over bed of spinach.

Shrimp Marinara

Sauté 1 clove garlic and 6 to 8 cleaned deveined large shrimp in 1 tablespoon olive oil. When shrimp turn pink, add ½ cup tomato sauce and cook 2 more minutes, or until tomato sauce is heated. Serve over 1 cup cooked spaghetti squash. (To cook spaghetti squash, cut squash in half, remove seeds, and place halves in glass baking dish in about ¼ inch of water. Bake at 350°F for 45 minutes, or until you can poke the squash skin easily with a fork.) Serve with a green side salad. (Allowable option: Top shrimp marinara with 2 tablespoons Parmesan cheese.)

Apricot Cod (4 servings)

Brew a strong cup of Numi White Nectar Tea (steep for 5 minutes). Pour cup of tea into skillet and let liquid come to a simmer. Place four 4-ounce pieces of cod into simmering tea. Season with garlic powder, sea salt, and white pepper to taste. Add 3 sliced apricots and cover pan with lid. Let fish steam for 10 to 15 minutes over medium heat until it easily flakes with a fork. Serve over spinach, next to steamed asparagus, or with a mixed green salad.

Fajita-Style Shrimp (2 servings)

Sauté 1 or 2 cloves chopped garlic and 15 cleaned deveined large shrimp in 1 tablespoon olive oil. As shrimp start to curl and change color, add 1 thinly sliced poblano chile pepper, 1 thinly sliced yellow bell pepper, and 1 chopped onion. Season with 1 tablespoon fajita seasoning, ¼ tsp (or more) cayenne pepper, and black pepper and sea salt to taste. Serve over a bed of spinach.

Cashew Chicken Curry (6 to 8 servings)

Sauté 2 chopped cloves garlic, 1 chopped onion, and 1 cup mushrooms with 3 pounds cubed chicken breast in 2 tablespoons coconut oil for 5 minutes. Season with 2 tablespoons curry powder, 1½ teaspoons paprika or cayenne pepper, and ¼ teaspoon cumin. Add ½ cup raw cashews and ¼ cup chopped cilantro. Cook for about 10 minutes. Add 1 can coconut milk, 1 (14-ounce) can stewed tomatoes, 1 (8-ounce) can tomato sauce, and 2 tablespoons lemon juice and stir well. Let simmer 30 to 40 minutes and serve in bowl over a generous handful of spinach.

Laura's Hearty Tuscan Soup (6 to 8 servings)

Sauté 3 cloves chopped garlic and 1 small chopped onion with 2 pounds ground chicken breast in 2 tablespoons olive oil for about 10 minutes (until chicken is nearly cooked). Add 1½ cups sliced mushrooms, 2 diced zucchinis, ½ teaspoon sea salt, and

½ teaspoon black pepper and cook for 5 minutes. Add 8 cups organic chicken broth and 1 can rinsed, drained cannellini beans and bring to a simmer. Add 1 cup fresh basil leaves. (Allowable option: 4 slices precooked turkey bacon, crumbled, and 1 cup organic half-and-half or cream or 1 cup So Delicious coconut milk if avoiding dairy.) Simmer 5 more minutes.

Bison-n-Kale Chipotle Chili (6 to 8 servings)

Sauté 4 cloves chopped garlic, 1 chopped onion, and 1 diced jalapeño chile pepper with 3 pounds ground bison in 3 tablespoons olive oil for 5 minutes. Add 1 bunch kale (cut into ½-inch-wide strips) and 2 cups sliced mushrooms. Season with ½ teaspoon cayenne, 2½ teaspoons minced chipotle chile pepper, 2 tablespoons cumin, 1 teaspoon black pepper, 2 teaspoons oregano, and 3 teaspoons onion powder. Cook for 3 to 5 minutes. Add 1 (28-ounce) can diced tomatoes, 1 (15-ounce) can tomato sauce, and 1 (15-ounce) can each drained and rinsed black and kidney beans. Bring to a simmer. Add 1 cleaned, finely chopped bunch of cilantro. Simmer chili for 15 minutes. Serve over a generous handful of spinach.

Turkey-Tomato Sauce (4 servings)

Sauté 1 clove garlic, 1 chopped onion, and 1 cup sliced mushrooms with 2 pounds ground white-meat turkey in 1 tablespoon olive oil. Season with Italian seasoning, sea salt, and black pepper to taste. Cook 5 minutes. Add 1 (16-ounce) jar store-bought marinara sauce. Serve atop a generous handful of spinach in a bowl, like a hearty soup.

Easy-Bake Options

Bake in glass if possible; no oil/greasing needed. If you use something else to bake, coat with olive-oil spray. Remember that most nonstick pots and pans are full of estrogenic chemicals.

Coconut Cinnamon Chicken

Place 4 chicken breasts in glass baking dish and pour 1 can coconut milk and ¼ cup lime juice over them. Sprinkle liberally with cinnamon (coating the top of each breast) and add 1 or 2 teaspoons xylitol and 3 tablespoons shredded coconut. Bake 30 minutes at 400°F. Makes 4 servings.

Baked Salmon & Red Swiss Chard

Dust 1 salmon fillet with a sprinkling of garlic powder and black pepper and bake at 450°F for 30 minutes, or until it flakes easily with a fork. While salmon is baking, cut cleaned red Swiss chard leaves into 1-inch-thick strips (include stalks). Sauté leaves in 1 teaspoon olive oil until they soften and just start to turn color (about 5 minutes). Season with sea salt, black pepper, garlic powder, and 1 teaspoon lemon juice.

Coconut Green Curry Chicken Meat Loaf

In a medium saucepan, combine 1 can coconut milk, 1 teaspoon green curry paste, and 2 tablespoons lime juice. Simmer about 15 minutes, or until the liquid thickens and reduces to about ⅓ cup. Set aside and let cool. In a large mixing bowl, add 1 tablespoon lime juice, ½ cup finely chopped fresh basil, ½ cup finely chopped fresh cilantro, ½ cup finely chopped unsalted peanuts, 1 cup shredded coconut, 2 tablespoons coconut oil, 1 tablespoon crushed red pepper flakes, and 2 teaspoons sea salt with 2 pounds ground chicken breast. Stir in cooled coconut milk mixture. Mix well and place in glass baking dish. Bake at 350°F for 30 minutes, or until chicken is completely cooked. Serve atop spinach or with Cucumber Pear Salad (page 279). Makes 6 servings.

Grass-Fed Meat Loaf

Sauté 3 chopped cloves garlic, 1 chopped onion, and 1½ cups sliced mushrooms in 2 tablespoons olive oil and let cool. In large mixing bowl, combine 2 pounds ground grass-fed beef, 3 cups ground broccoli (use food processor to finely chop broccoli), 1 teaspoon black pepper, 2 teaspoons sea salt, 1 tablespoon prepared mustard, 1 tablespoon Worcestershire sauce, and ½ cup almond flour. Mix together well, using your hands. Place mixture in glass baking dish and bake uncovered at 350°F for 45 to 60 minutes. Makes 6 servings. Variation: Make this mixture into **Grass-Fed Meat Muffins,** an excellent snack. Simply put mixture into muffin tins, filling each nearly to the top. Bake for 20 minutes at 350°F. Makes 12 muffins.

Other Allowable Options

Cheesy Fish Casserole

Toast 1 slice hemp or sprouted-grain bread and crumble into crumbs; set aside. Mix 4 ounces canned or fresh cooked fish (salmon, flounder, tuna, etc.) with 1 cup chopped broccoli, 1 egg, 1 cup milk or unsweetened almond milk, 2 tablespoons lemon juice, and sea salt and pepper to taste. (Allowable option: ¼ cup grated low-fat Swiss or other low-fat cheese.) Stir in bread crumbs. Place mixture in glass baking dish and bake at 375°F for 15 minutes.

Sausage & Pepper Stir-Fry

Sauté 1 clove chopped garlic in 1 tablespoon olive oil with 4 ounces sliced chicken or turkey sausage, 1½ cups chopped bell pepper, and 1 chopped onion. Serve over a bed of spinach.

NOTES FOR EASY-BAKE OPTIONS

- If not following low-insulin protocol, it is okay to add 1 serving (⅓ to ½ cup or 4 to 6 bites) of an Allowable high-fiber starch or a piece of Optimal fruit, if not otherwise listed.
- Green veggies should be eaten liberally, and it is fine to go over recommended amounts above for any nonstarchy vegetable or to serve spinach or green salad alongside any option.

Quick and Tasty High-Fiber Starch/Carb Options

Tapas-Style Chickpeas

Warm 1 to 2 teaspoons olive oil in small frying pan. Add 2 cups cooked or 1 can rinsed and drained chickpeas, ½ teaspoon garlic powder, and both sea salt and hot paprika to taste. Cook until "toasted."

Lentil Salad

Mix 2 cups cooked or 1 can rinsed and drained lentils with 1 diced cucumber, 1 diced tomato or bell pepper, 3 chopped scallions, and both sea salt and pepper to taste. (For an Allowable option, add ⅓ cup feta cheese.) Makes 2 servings.

Spicy Black Beans

Place 2 cups cooked or 1 can rinsed and drained black beans in small saucepan with ¼ cup chicken broth, ¼ teaspoon cayenne pepper, ¼ teaspoon minced chipotle chile pepper, and sea salt and pepper to taste. Over medium-low heat, warm beans, mashing them into a paste (refried beans–style). Serves 4.

Hemp or Sprouted-Grain Garlic Toast

Drizzle 1 slice of bread with mixture of 1 teaspoon olive oil, ¼ teaspoon garlic powder, and ¼ teaspoon sea salt. Toast in broiler about 3 to 5 minutes.

SNACKS AND DESSERTS

- 2 hard-boiled eggs and ½ cup blueberries
- Celery or carrot sticks with 2 teaspoons natural nut butter
- Apple with ¼ cup nuts or 2 teaspoons nut butter
- 1 can sardines and ½ cup raspberries
- 1 can salmon, trout, or tuna and 1 pear
- 3 ounces sliced turkey and 1 green apple
- ½ bison or grass-fed beef burger and 1 small sliced tomato
- ½ slice veggie quiche
- Ultimate You Lean Bar, PaleoBar, or Biogenesis Ultra Low Carb bar
- 3 or 4 Slentiva chews (www.bodybyhardware.com)
- 4 Brain Power Sours (www.bodybyhardware.com)
- ½ avocado, pit removed, hole filled with balsamic vinegar; sea salt and pepper to taste; eat with a spoon, scooping out avocado flesh from outer skin, mixing each bit in the vinegar
- 1 or 2 Grass-Fed Meat Muffins (page 284) with 1 cup cucumber slices
- Bell pepper slices dipped in ½ cup Guacamole (page 288)
- Soft Cinnamon Apples (opposite)
- 1 Cocoa Coconut PB Protein No-Bake Cookie (opposite) with 1 cup Numi Chocolate Puerh Tea (optional, page 167)

- 1 or 2 Spinach Timbales (below) and ¼ cup cashews
- ¼ cup Not-Granola (below)
- ¼ cup Spicy Nut Mix (page 288)

Optimal Snacks

Soft Cinnamon Apples

Slice and sauté 1 tart apple in 1 tablespoon water. As apple softens, sprinkle liberally with cinnamon and 1 teaspoon xylitol. Cook 3 to 5 more minutes. Place in small bowl and top with 2 teaspoons chunky almond butter.

Cocoa Coconut PB Protein No-Bake Cookies

In medium mixing bowl, stir together 4 scoops Ultimate Whey, 1½ cups whole rolled oats, 2 tablespoons cocoa powder, ½ cup shredded coconut, 3 teaspoons Truvia (about 4 packets), ¾ cup natural chunky peanut butter, 1 teaspoon natural vanilla extract, and 1 cup unsweetened chocolate almond milk. Spoon onto wax paper in ¼-cup "balls" and refrigerate for at least 1 hour before serving. Serving is 1 cookie; recipe makes 6 to 8 cookies.

Spinach Timbales

Sauté 1 clove chopped garlic and 1 chopped onion in 1 tablespoon olive oil; set aside. In large bowl, mix 6 eggs with ½ cup milk or unsweetened almond milk, a dash of nutmeg, ½ teaspoon salt, and ½ teaspoon cracked black pepper. Completely thaw 2 pounds frozen spinach and press out all water (equals 2 cups spinach). Add onion and spinach to egg mixture and stir well. (Allowable option: Add ½ cup feta cheese.) Spoon mixture into muffin tin, filling each cup about ¾ full. Bake for 30 minutes at 350°F. Store extra timbales in refrigerator for up to 1 week. Serves 10 to 12.

Not-Granola

Mix 1 cup each almonds, hazelnuts, and pecans with ½ cup large flaked coconut, 2 teaspoons cinnamon, a dash of nutmeg, 1 tablespoon xylitol, and 2 tablespoons coconut oil. (Solid coconut oil softens nicely in a warm water bath; pour off liquid and measure.) Spread onto cookie sheet and bake at 400°F for 10 to 15 minutes. Serves 8.

Spicy Nut Mix

Mix together 1 cup Brazil nuts, 1 cup pistachios, 1 cup cashews, ½ teaspoon sea salt, ½ teaspoon Italian seasoning blend, ½ teaspoon garlic powder, ¼ teaspoon cayenne pepper, and 2 tablespoons olive oil. Spread onto cookie sheet and bake at 400°F for 10 to 15 minutes. Serves 8.

Guacamole

In a large bowl, mash 2 large peeled and pitted avocados. Add 1 diced Roma tomato, 1 finely chopped jalapeño chile pepper (cleaned, with seeds and stem removed), 3 tablespoons finely chopped red onion, 2 tablespoons finely chopped cilantro, and 1 tablespoon lime juice. Season with ½ teaspoon garlic powder and ½ teaspoon onion powder. Add salt and freshly ground black pepper to taste. Serves 4.

Allowable Snack Options

- 1 cup plain yogurt or cottage cheese with berries, 10 almonds, or ¼ cup Not-Granola (page 287)
- Cleaned bell pepper with stem removed, cut into 4 large wedges; spread with 2 ounces goat cheese and add cracked black pepper to taste
- ½ scoop whey protein powder mixed with 1 teaspoon Ultimate Fiber and ½ cup coconut water; shake and drink

Allowable Sweet Snacks and Dessert-Craving Busters

- 2 ounces dark chocolate
- **Coconut Cream Pie:** Mix ½ cup low-fat Greek yogurt with 3 tablespoons unsweetened shredded coconut and 1 packet Truvia.
- **Pumpkin Custard:** Mix ½ cup organic canned pumpkin with 1 tablespoon xylitol, ½ scoop Ultimate Whey Vanilla, 1½ tablespoons unsweetened vanilla almond milk, ½ teaspoon (or more to taste) cinnamon, and a dash of nutmeg.
- **Warm Berry Compote:** Warm ¾ cup frozen berries in microwave until thawed and soft (about 90 seconds). Stir in 1 packet Truvia and ½ scoop Ultimate Whey, sprinkle with cinnamon, and top with about 10 almonds or 2 tablespoons Not-Granola (page 287).

- **Chocolate Walnut Pudding:** Mix ½ cup low-fat Greek yogurt with ½ scoop Ultimate Chocolate Whey Protein. Top with 2 tablespoons chopped walnuts.

- **Coconut Ice Cream:** Mix 1 bag frozen berries, 1 cup shredded coconut, 1 can light coconut milk, 1 tablespoon xylitol, and 1 teaspoon almond or vanilla extract in blender or food processor. Freeze in glass Pyrex bowl. Serving size: ½ cup.

Allowable Indulgent Desserts

All Ultimate You dessert recipes courtesy of Colorado-based caterer/cook Thadd Hollis—the Ultimate You Recipe Makeover Man!

Flourless Chocolate Cake with Xylitol

Preheat oven to 375°F. Butter 8-inch round cake pan. Chop 7 ounces bittersweet chocolate (60 to 65 percent cocoa) into small pieces; melt in double boiler. Add 7 ounces organic unsalted butter (softened) and a pinch of salt. Stir with a heat-resistant spatula until smooth.

Separate 4 room-temperature eggs and reserve whites and yolks in 2 bowls. Add ½ cup xylitol to egg yolks; beat until pale in color. Add in the chocolate/butter mixture.

In another bowl, beat egg whites until soft peaks form. Gradually add another ½ cup xylitol to beaten egg whites until mixture is smooth and shiny and stiff peaks form. Fold one-third of the egg-white mixture into the chocolate mixture to soften. Continue to gently fold in the remaining egg-white mixture until incorporated (be careful not to overmix).

Pour the batter into the prepared pan and bake for 35 to 40 minutes, or until a toothpick inserted into the center comes out clean. Let the cake rest at room temperature for 10 minutes before turning it out of the pan. Serve warm, at room temperature, or cold. Serves 6 to 8.

Roasted Figs with Gorgonzola

Preheat oven to 400°F. Rub 12 ripe figs all over with 2 tablespoons extra-virgin olive oil. Make a single cut lengthwise in each fig, cutting only halfway through; set aside. In a small bowl, crumble ¼ cup gorgonzola cheese (for a lower-fat option, use low-fat feta cheese) and mix with 2 tablespoons coarsely chopped walnuts; place about 1 teaspoon mixture into each fig. Bake about 10 minutes, or until figs are soft and caramelized. Serve warm. Serves 6.

Fresh Fruit & Mint in Red Wine

Rinse and dry 1 pound of cherries, strawberries, or peaches. Stem strawberries, stem and pit cherries, or cut peaches into wedges. Place fruit in a shallow bowl and toss with ¼ cup red wine and ¼ cup mint leaves. Place in refrigerator to chill for 30 minutes to 2 hours prior to serving. Serves 6.

Resources

Where to Get Products We Recommend

www.betterbydrbrooke.com: paraben-free cosmetics, deodorants, and skin care

www.bodybyhardware.com: exercise balls, foam rollers, jump ropes, The Stick, Polar heart-rate monitors, exercise bands, exercise mats, adjustable aerobic steps, PowerBlocks, weight bench; paraben-free cosmetics, deodorants, skin care, supplements, DVDs, and other supportive tools

www.doultonusa.com: high-quality water filters

www.fitnessmart.com: Gullick II tape measure

www.grasslandbeef.com: grass-fed, organic beef shipped to your home

www.hightechhealth.com: high-quality water filters

www.lanisimpson.com: paraben-free cosmetics, deodorants, and skin care

www.lavanila.com: Lavanila natural deodorant

www.nowfoods.com: Now brand liquid stevia (also available at most health-food stores)

www.numitea.com: Numi brand tea (also available at Whole Foods and many health-food stores)

www.performbetter.com: exercise balls, foam rollers, jump ropes, The Stick, Polar heart-rate monitors, exercise bands, exercise mats, and adjustable aerobic steps

www.powerblock.com: PowerBlocks, weight bench

www.sallyhansennaturalbeauty.com: paraben-free cosmetics

www.sephora.com: Lavanila natural deodorant

www.tropicaltraditions.com: source for organic, extra-virgin coconut oil and coconut oil–based products

www.vitalchoice.com: wild seafood and other organic products

Where to Find Supplements, Bars & Protein Shakes

www.biogenesis.com: Biogenesis UltraLean low carb bars

www.bodybyhardware.com: Hardware, Designs for Health, Biogenesis products, and more

www.charlespoliquin.com: Poliquin Performance Products

www.designsforhealth.com: Designs for Health products

www.jayrobb.com: Jay Robb whey protein, also available at Vitamin Shoppe, Whole Foods, and other health-food stores

Books We Recommend

Achieving Victory Over a Toxic World by Mark Schauss, MBA, DB

Advanced Nutrition and Human Metabolism by James L. Groff and Sareen S. Gropper

Core Performance: The Revolutionary Workout Program to Transform Your Body and Your Life by Mark Verstegen

Dr. Brady's Healthy Revolution: What You Need to Know to Stay Healthy in a Sick World by Dr. David M. Brady

The Edge Effect: Achieve Total Health and Longevity with the Balanced Brain Advantage by Eric Braverman, MD

Facts and Fallacies of Fitness by Mel C. Siff, PhD

Functional Metabolism: Regulation and Adaptation by Kenneth B. Storey

Fundamentals of Naturopathic Endocrinology by Michael Friedman

The 150 Healthiest Foods on Earth: The Surprising, Unbiased Truth about What You Should Eat and Why by Jonny Bowden, PhD, CNS

Physiology of Sport and Exercise by Jack H. Wilmore and David L. Costill

Power Healing: Use the New Integrated Medicine to Cure Yourself by Leo Galland, MD

Robert Crayhon's Nutrition Made Simple by Robert Crayhon, MS

Russian Sports Restoration and Massage by Michael Yessis, PhD

Strength Training for Women by Lori Incledon

Supertraining by Mel C. Siff, PhD

Total Heart Rate Training: Customize and Maximize Your Workout Using a Heart Rate Monitor by Joe Friel

Ultimate Back Fitness and Performance by Stuart McGill, PhD

The Whole Soy Story: The Dark Side of America's Favorite Health Food by Kaayla T Daniel, PhD, CCN

The Women's Health Big Book of Exercises by Adam Campbell, MS, CSCS

Why Do I Still Have Thyroid Symptoms When My Lab Tests Are Normal?: A Revolutionary Breakthrough in Understanding Hashimoto's Disease and Hypothyroidism by Datis Kharrazian, DHSc, DC, MS

Yen and Jaffe's Reproductive Endocrinology: Physiology, Pathophysiology, and Clinical Management edited by Jerome Strauss and Robert Barbieri

Informative Web Sites

www.bastyr.edu: site for Bastyr University (Seattle)

www.betterbydrbrooke.com: site for Dr. Brooke's private practice in New York City

www.bodybyhardware.com: nutrition and exercise articles, blog, workouts, supplements, and more from Joe Dowdell and Dr. Brooke Kalanick

www.coreperformance.com: excellent resource for training and nutrition

www.cosmeticsdatabase.com: site for searching cosmetic ingredient safety

www.functionalmedicine.org: site for the Institute for Functional Medicine

www.naturopathic.org: site for the American Association of Naturopathic Physicians

www.peakperformancenyc.com: site for Joe Dowdell's personal training facility in New York City

www.westonaprice.org: information on food, farming, and diet research

Informative Web Sites

www.bastyr.edu: site for Bastyr University (Seattle)

www.betterbydrbrooke.com: site for Dr. Brooke's private practice in New York City

www.bodybyhardware.com: nutrition and exercise articles, blog, workouts, supplements, and more from Joe Dowdell and Dr. Brooke Kalanick

www.coreperformance.com: excellent resource for training and nutrition

www.cosmeticsdatabase.com: site for searching cosmetic ingredient safety

www.functionalmedicine.org: site for the Institute for Functional Medicine

www.naturopathic.org: site for the American Association of Naturopathic Physicians

www.peakperformancenyc.com: site for Joe Dowdell's personal training facility in New York City

www.westonaprice.org: information on food, farming, and diet research

Acknowledgments

Thank you to my parents, Lynda and Joseph Dowdell, because without their constant love, support, and encouragement over the course of my life I would never be in the position I am today; and to my sisters, Melissa and Kristen, whom I love and admire very much.

To my mentors, Charles Poliquin, Paul Chek, Tom Purvis, and the late Dr. Mel Siff, each of whom has had a profound impact on my thought process as a fitness professional. Their leadership has helped me improve the lifestyle and aesthetics of my clients as well as the performance of my athletes.

To the other influential doctors, strength coaches, and fitness professionals who over the years have helped influence my development as a fitness professional, including Dr. John Berardi, Dr. Leo Galland, Mark Verstegen, Mike Boyle, Darryl Eto, Dave Tate, Eric Cressey, Mike Robertson, Paul Robbins, Alwyn Cosgrove, Joe Gomes, Gray Cook, Nick Winkleman, and Greg Roskoff.

To my literary agent, David Vigliano, who convinced me that I needed to write a book and helped me find a home at Rodale.

To my editor, Shannon Welch, who spent countless hours making sure that this book came to fruition.

To Steve Murphy, my client and friend, who offered me so much helpful information during this whole process.

To my coauthor, Dr. Brooke Kalanick, whose intelligence, work ethic, and dedication to her profession (and this book) never ceases to amaze me. And without her contributions to this book, it would not be the same end result.

To all the staff, trainers, and clients at Peak Performance who make me want to go to work every day. I love what I do because of you. And especially to Kindra Hanson, Tim Davis, Jay Wright, and Matt McGorry, for offering tremendous support while I was pursuing this dream.

And to my little girl (and official mascot of Peak Performance)—my rottweiler Sky who brings lots of happiness and laughs into my life.

—Joe

There would be no *Ultimate You* without Shannon Welch, our editor at Rodale, who is forever a rock star to me! Thank you for the countless late-night hours you gave us. To everyone at Rodale and Vigliano Associates for their help, and to Steve Murphy for your guidance. And many thanks to Julia VanTine, whose expertise helped us make extremely complex ideas accessible to every woman and helped me become a better writer.

Thank you to all of my functional-medicine teachers, including Dr. Datis Kharrazian, Dr. Leo Galland, and Dr. David Brady. To the innovators of fitness, including Charles Poliquin. I appreciate the amazing and thoughtful information you are putting out into the world. And to my friend and colleague, Jade Teta, ND, for teaching me so much and for helping me turn a personal interest in exercise and nutrition into an amazing career that I love.

Thank you to my patients—you teach me something new every day, and I truly appreciate your support and patience this past year.

To my wonderful friends: Taryn, for never letting me get away with less than my best—you always make me feel better, no matter what; Darcy, for your friendship and your fabulous talents—your design help has been invaluable; Lorraine, for your constant support and level head—you keep me sane; and Shirin, who manages to be my makeup artist, stylist, photographer, and friend all at once. You all mean the world to me.

To my family, thank you, and I love you all: Jessica, Miluše, McKenzie, Holly and the Kaleczycs, Sally, Laura, Gary, Megan, Emily, Greg, and Miriam. To my brother Dustin, for always being there when I need you. And last but not least, to my dad— without his unwavering support and belief in me, none of the dreams I've ever had would be a reality.

Words can't say how much I appreciate everyone at Peak Performance. Thank you for all the support you've given me this past year—and thank you for cheering me on as I push the prowler! I am so grateful for you all. Special thanks to Brendan, Rob, Mark, Matt, and Tim for your friendship and encouragement.

To my Joes: First, to Joe Dowdell (the one I work with). You are hands-down one of the best and smartest trainers I've ever met. Your commitment to learning and excellence in training impresses me every day. I can't wait for women everywhere to be "trained" by you through our book! Thanks for all your hard work as we've made Hardware and *Ultimate You* a reality—looking forward to all we'll accomplish together!

Finally, to Joe Larson (the one I live with). Thank you for moving to New York with me and for dreaming very big dreams with me. I love you so much, and you make me feel like I can do anything. Thanks for being my anchor every day, for tolerating me when I stress out (sorry!), for never letting me give up, for making me a better person . . . and for making me laugh every day since I've known you.

—Brooke

Finally, to Joe Larson (the one I live with). Thank you for moving to New York with me and for dreaming very big dreams with me. I love you so much, and you make me feel like I can do anything. Thanks for being my anchor every day, for tolerating me when I stress out (sorry!), for never letting me give up, for making me a better person . . . and for making me laugh every day since I've known you.

—Brooke

Index

Boldface page references indicate photographs. Underscored references indicate boxed text.